Finding out wh[...]*test has transformed my life. For the first time in 13 years I'm pain free.* – Denise Lewis, Olympic gold medal winner and star of the hit TV show *Strictly Come Dancing*

This book beautifully explains how food allergy and intolerance is responsible for much widespread chronic poor health today. As well as being an invaluable tool for those wanting to manage their condition, this is required reading for every clinician. – Maureen Jenkins, Trustee of Allergy UK and from Sussex Allergy Advice

I feel so much better. Nothing like as tired. I have no bloating. My eczema is a lot better. And I've even lost a couple of pounds. – Liza

I've definitely lost weight and am much less bloated. People have noticed I've got my waist back and I'm in trousers I haven't worn for years. My constipation has completely gone. I used to use my inhaler four times a day, now I don't use it at all. Overall I feel so much better. – Katie

My energy is better and I'm more alert. My IBS has been better and I have a lot less trapped wind. I used to get tired after a meal – and I would get the feeling of still being hungry. I don't get that so much anymore. I would often get more pain after eating. That's reduced too. Overall I feel really good. – Leanne

I can't tell you how much better I feel. I'm 100 per cent. Having the food intolerance test has been the best thing I've done. It has transformed my health. I have lost the entire 140lb (64kg) that I'd put on over the past three years. I wish I'd done it sooner! – Rebecca

Within a week of cutting all dairy products from his diet, my hyperactive seven-year-old was less excitable, more settled, and could concentrate better so he is now doing much better in school. His chronic insomnia has gone and he now sleeps through the night. He doesn't need the steroid medication for his asthma any more. – Iain's mum

Within a week I was going to the loo every two days (instead of weekly), my tummy was gone and I was down to a size 12 from a size 16. My lethargy was caused by the yeasty foods I ate. I've gone from 156lb (about 70kg) to 129lb (58kg), and look so much trimmer now. – Joanne

Within a couple of days of cutting these foods out of my diet, I began to feel better. My head felt clearer, my energy levels and sinusitis improved and even my rheumatoid arthritis pain eased considerably. After ten years of frequent and severe headaches and migraines, I am pleased to say that these have also dramatically reduced. – Alison

Life is now free of pain and medication and I have complete mobility. I am amazed at the difference in my quality of life simply by making such simple adjustments. – John

About ten days after starting the diet I noticed I was less tired in the morning. Now I'm not tired at all when I wake up. I have loads more energy, I'm less bored, I'm concentrating better and I feel a lot happier. I'm getting on better at school and concentrating better in class. I'm also doing more activities and sports, I'm a lot calmer than I used to be and I'm not getting into trouble at school anymore. I feel more positive about my future. I'm going to stay on the diet for life. It's brilliant! – Liam (14)

I started feeling better after one week on the diet. For three years I had suffered with joint pain and swelling in my hands, ankles and arms, shooting pains in my arms and legs, fluid retention, extreme fatigue, uncontrollable food cravings, heartburn, chronic skin rashes and heart palpitations despite taking several prescription medications. By seven weeks later all of my symptoms had gone and I had stopped all my medication. I also lost 15lb (7kg). – Cathy

My life-long lethargy has lifted, I've lost all my constipation, bloatedness and pain. I am simply delighted. – Sandra

HIDDEN FOOD ALLERGIES

PATRICK HOLFORD AND DR JAMES BRALY

PIATKUS

✥ Visit the Piatkus website!

Piatkus publishes a wide range of best-selling fiction and non-fiction, including books on health, mind, body & spirit, sex, self-help, cookery, biography and the paranormal.

If you want to:
- read descriptions of our popular titles
- buy our books over the Internet
- take advantage of our special offers
- enter our monthly competition
- learn more about your favourite Piatkus authors

VISIT OUR WEBSITE AT: www.piatkus.co.uk

Copyright © 2005 by Patrick Holford and Dr James Braly

First published in Great Britain in 2005 by
Piatkus Books Ltd
5 Windmill Street, London W1T 2JA
email: info@piatkus.co.uk

Reprinted 2005, 2006, 2007

The moral right of the authors has been asserted

A catalogue record for this book is available from the British Library

ISBN 978 0 7499 2602 1

Edited by Barbara Kiser
Text design by Paul Saunders

This book has been printed on paper manufactured
with respect for the environment using wood from
managed sustainable resources

Typeset by Phoenix Photosetting, Chatham, Kent
Printed and bound in Great Britain by Mackays of Chatham, Chatham, Kent

Contents

Introduction

Finding and Losing Your Hidden Food Allergies

HOW ARE YOU FEELING, right at this moment? The odds are that it's well below your potential for pain-free, symptom-free, high-energy living – and all for a simple reason. You are eating or drinking something that doesn't suit you.

Your reaction to what you eat may not be immediate or severe. But it could be insidiously adding to your burden of unwellness, with the potential to tip over into chronic health problems such as irritable bowel syndrome, migraine, chronic fatigue or asthma.

Of course, there are other allergens – airborne substances such as pollen, or dust mites or cats' dander (flakes of the animals' skin). Chemicals in food, household products or the environment can be culprits, too. The most common, however, is food.

Officially, an estimated one in three of us have an allergy, according to a survey by the Royal College of Physicians.[1] But this could be a serious underestimate. In Europe, allergy is considered to be the number one chronic illness. And in one survey of 3,300 adults, 43 per cent said that they experienced adverse reactions to food.[2] In another, 70 per cent of people suffering from a wide range of chronic illnesses discussed in this book, who had failed to respond to conventional treatment, found relief from their symptoms by identifying their food allergies and avoiding those foods.[3] Almost a quarter obtained 100 per cent relief!

In our experience, the vast majority of people have no idea their health problems may be related to eating specific foods. Most people's food allergies are truly hidden from them.

The truth is that the majority of people, including you, are likely to suffer for years not only not knowing they have an allergy – but also, not knowing how to treat it by identifying which foods they react to and how to regain their tolerance to those foods. Our personal stories are a case in point.

■ We've been there...

I (Patrick Holford) suffered throughout my childhood and adolescence from migraines, sinus problems and ear infections. I saw countless doctors and specialists, had my adenoids and tonsils removed, and had two sinus operations, numerous courses of antibiotics and many nights of excruciating pain from migraines – only to discover that I was allergic to milk and yeast.

I (James Braly) also suffered from severe, disabling migraines as a child – so severe that my left eye crossed and the pupil dilated. It was only as an adult that I finally discovered I was allergic to dairy products. Gluten grains – wheat, rye and barley products in particular – were also causing nasal congestion, skin rashes when I ran long distances, extreme bloating and sleepiness after eating, and on rare occasions muscle spasms in my air passages, causing them to temporarily close shut and my breathing to become extremely difficult. Ironically, wheat and cow's milk were my favourite food groups throughout my childhood and adolescence. I went for many years without suspecting either to be the underlying causes of my symptoms. Now, without dairy and the gluten grains in my diet, I remain free of migraines, nasal congestion, hives and breathing problems.

Your symptoms may be more or less severe than ours, and caused by factors other than food allergies. Chances are, however, that food intolerances or allergies are adding to your burden, and in many cases, are proving to be the main cause of any health problems. This constitutes unnecessary suffering, and as we don't want you to have to struggle with it any longer, we have written this book to guide you through the maze of discovering which foods make you ill and what to eat instead. We'll let you know about the amazing scientific advances that mean you can now identify food allergies from a pinprick of blood using a simple home test kit.

What's more, we'll explain why you become intolerant to certain foods by revealing the underlying causes of most food allergies, and how to eliminate these causes and thereby reduce your allergic potential. We'll explain how to 'desensitise' yourself to foods you're allergic to so you can eat them once more, a process that usually takes just three months.

Some types of allergies, of course, are for life. If you have this kind, you can't desensitise yourself completely – but you can reduce the severity of your allergic symptoms using natural, drug-free methods, and we will show you a range.

■ How to use this book

But first, here's an overview of what you'll find in this book. Chapter 1 helps you discover if your health problems are likely to be caused by something you are eating and, if so, whether that is triggering a food allergy, food sensitivity or intolerance. Chapter 2 explains the two main types of food allergy: immediate-onset 'IgE based' allergy, and the much more prevalent delayed or hidden 'IgG-based' food allergy. Chapter 3 runs through the most common health problems associated with food allergy.

If you've got children, Chapter 4 lets you know how to prevent and solve childhood allergies, and the common health problems they cause. Chapter 5 goes through the top 20 common food allergens. Chapter 6 tells you how to identify which foods you are allergic to, while Chapter 7 explains the basis for correcting the underlying causes that lead to allergy in the first place. Finally, Chapter 8 gives you a clear action plan for relief from food allergies, then segues into the appendices. Here, you'll find useful information on food families (so if you're allergic to one food, you can make informed choices about eating any of its 'relatives'), a symptom score chart, and detailed information on the severe gluten allergy, coeliac disease.

Throughout, our promise to you is this: we will help you improve your health by finding out which foods suit you and which foods trigger an allergic reaction, show you how to desensitise yourself to most all of those foods, and give you the know-how to achieve *permanent* allergy relief. And all without the need for medication or restrictive diets.

Wishing you the best of allergy-free health!

Patrick Holford and Dr James Braly

1

Is What You Eat Making You Ill?

IF **YOU HAVE** niggling or serious health problems that come and go, or are worse after eating certain foods, better on holiday when your diet is different, or unresponsive to conventional medical treatment, now is a good moment to question whether something you are eating is making you ill.

Most major health problems – diabetes, heart disease, even Alzheimer's and most types of cancer – are now recognised as primarily diet related. So why shouldn't headaches, anxiety, digestive problems, joint aches, fatigue or whatever it is you are suffering from be diet related?

In most cases, they are. There may, of course, be other contributory factors; but finding out which foods suit you and which foods don't can make a massive difference to how you feel.

■ Three typical stories

To show how this works, we asked Britain's most watched breakfast television franchise, GMTV – for which Patrick is nutrition expert – to give us three volunteers with different health problems who had had no relief from conventional medicine, and to allow us three weeks to find out whether food was making them ill.

Liza, the first, had suffered from eczema since early childhood. She also felt tired a lot of the time, and suffered from occasional bloating and weight fluctuations. She kept her eczema under control with a cortisone-based cream, but her hands were still crinkly and sore. She also drank coffee or caffeinated drinks throughout the day to keep her awake.

The second, Katie, had all the classic symptoms of irritable bowel syndrome – bloating, abdominal pain, constipation and occasional diarrhoea. She also had asthma and used an inhaler several times each day. She had gained 28lb (nearly 13kg) in weight and gone up two dress sizes. Her doctor had given her Fybogel, a type of fibre, but it didn't help. She suspected that she was reacting to certain foods but didn't know what.

The third was Leanne. Chronically tired, Leanne thought wheat made her worse and had avoided it. But she still felt exhausted most of the time, and on top of that had migraines, a poor sex drive and digestive problems. She'd been tested for thyroid problems and glandular fever, but there was no conventional medical diagnosis or treatment for her condition.

We tested each volunteer for food allergy with a simple home-test kit using a pinprick of blood. Liza, we found, was strongly allergic to dairy products; Katie was allergic to yeast, almonds and cashews; and Leanne had multiple food allergies. As well as giving general advice about healthy eating, they were each given some specific supplements such as multivitamins, digestive enzymes, probiotics and glutamine (more on this in Chapter 6). Liza was advised to quit all caffeine.

Here's what happened, in their own words, three weeks later.

Liza: *I feel so much better. Nothing like as tired. I am really surprised at how easy I found it to cut out the caffeine, and I have more energy, not less. The milk avoidance itself wasn't so difficult, but I was amazed to find out how many foods had hidden milk; so it took a week to discover what I could and couldn't have. Overall it's been fine. I have no bloating. My skin is a lot better. I have no sores or cuts. I have lost a couple of pounds.*

Katie: *People have noticed I've got my waist back. I'm in trousers I haven't worn for years. I am much less bloated. I've had very few stomach cramps. I've definitely lost weight. I went out for dinner at an Indian restaurant and had no reaction. I'm also using my inhaler much less. I used to use my inhaler four times a day, now none. One day I inadvertently had some muesli with almonds, one of my allergy foods. I felt itchy after that. My constipation has completely gone. Used to go once a week and suffer stomach pains in between. Now I go every day. Overall I feel so much better.*

Leanne: *My energy is better and I'm more alert. My IBS has been OK, better, not dramatic, although I do have a lot less wind pain. I don't get so tired. I used to get tired after a meal – I would get the feeling of still being hungry. I don't get that so much any more. I would often get more pain after eating. That's reduced too. Overall I feel really good but there's still room for improvement.*

These three cases show how important it is to pinpoint precisely what you're allergic to. Simply put, a food allergy means your immune system is producing antibodies designed to attack certain proteins you eat, causing symptoms. And that's what was happening to Liza when she consumed dairy products.

We'll be exploring allergies in depth in the next chapter, but first let's take a look at the other ways food can affect your well-being.

▪ When it's not an allergy...

Food intolerance

As we've seen, Liza coped with exhaustion by guzzling coffee and caffeinated drinks. Little did she know that the caffeine was actually making her more tired. Some foods or drinks knock your system out of balance, and two of the big culprits are sugar and caffeine (also present in tea). The more of these you eat or drink, the more resistant you may become to their effects, resulting in rebound exhaustion. This is an intolerance.

There are other kinds of food intolerance which we define as a non-immunological response to a food – that is, you get symptoms, but there's no observable or measurable immune reaction. The most common example is intolerance of lactose – milk sugar, found in cow's milk – which happens in people who lack adequate supplies of the enzyme lactase, which is needed to digest it. This kind of intolerance means milk is hard to digest – a very different thing from an allergy to cow's milk, where the immune reaction can cause inflammation (in Liza's case, resulting in eczema). Lactose intolerance and milk allergy do often go hand in hand, however.

Food/chemical sensitivity

Some people – often those who also have food allergies – are especially sensitive to certain chemicals added to food. Their symptoms can be very similar to allergic reactions, and may include hives or urticaria, which are eruptions of itchy bumps on the skin. In children with chronic hives, sensitivity to a food additive such as food colourings, preservatives, emulsifiers or taste enhancers is a possible cause. A recent double-blind, placebo-controlled study showed that 3 out of every 4 children with chronic hives greatly improved within 2 weeks on a food additive-free diet, while half the children had complete relief by 6 months.[4] If, however, you or your child suffers from hives which don't improve on avoiding additives, we recommend that you investigate food allergies as a probable cause.

Four common additives that often provoke symptoms are:

- **MSG (monosodium glutamate)** (E621), a taste enhancer found in Chinese food, much of restaurant fast food and many tinned or packaged foods. Symptoms can include nausea, vomiting, headaches and dizziness.

- **Sulphites/metasulphites/metabisulphites** (E221 and 223, for example), used to maintain freshness, are common in factory-prepared foods and white wines, and often added to potatoes, avocados, shellfish, greens and vegetables in restaurant salad bars. Asthmatics may have severe reactions to sulfites. Sulphite sensitivity may be associated with a molybdenum trace mineral deficiency.

■ **Tartrazine** (E102) is used widely as a food colouring and is known to cause hyperactivity, migraines and asthmatic attacks. It also depletes the body of vitamin B6 and zinc.

■ **BHA** (E320) is used as a preservative, especially in foods containing fats, and confectionery and meats. It can cause hives and other skin reactions.

■ **Inulin**, extracted from artichokes, and its chemical cousin oligofructose are now added to an increasing number of industrially processed foods, such as sweets, drinks, yoghurt, ice cream, chocolate, butter and breakfast cereals. It can cause allergy-like symptoms, such as breathing difficulties, in susceptible people.

While we won't be covering chemical sensitivity any further than this, we recommend that everyone avoids food containing these additives as much as possible.

Food poisoning

Food poisoning – characterised by nausea, vomiting and diarrhoea – is a widespread and serious problem with a number of causes. Some plants and animals are simply unsafe for human consumption. For example, the 'death cap' family of mushrooms can trigger severe or even fatal poisoning. A more common source is spoiled or improperly cooked food. Chicken, for instance, can be rife with 'bad' bacteria such as salmonella.

In Britain alone there are 100,000 reported cases of food poisoning a year, but probably over 20 times that number go unreported, often because the symptoms don't always develop immediately and affected people fail to realise it's caused by something they ate, or don't go to the doctor. People often assume they are allergic to shellfish, for example, when they may have no allergy but have had a bout of food poisoning.

Nutritional deficiency

Another possible reason why what you're eating is making you ill is simply that it's poor-quality food, lacking in nutrients. Say you live on processed food and don't consume much fruit, vegetables or wholefoods (that is, beans, lentils, nuts, seeds, brown rice or wholegrain breads and pastas). If that's you, you may find yourself feeling tired and unwell because you're simply not getting the vitamins and minerals your mind and body need.

We recommend a good all-round diet and basic supplement programme for everybody to ensure optimum nutrition, and to make you less prone to developing an allergy (see Chapter 8).

■ Are you suffering from a hidden food allergy?

We've now looked at a number of food-related reactions. But what if your problems with a food or foods don't match up? Let's examine the classic symptoms of a food allergy now, to discover whether this is what you're suffering from.

The symptoms below are the most common signs of increased likelihood for allergy. Score 1 point for each 'yes' answer.

Your Instant Allergy Check

☐ Are you chronically tired?

☐ Can you gain weight in hours?

☐ Do you get bloated after eating?

☐ Do you suffer from diarrhoea or constipation?

☐ Do you suffer from abdominal pain?

☐ Do you sometimes get really sleepy after eating?

☐ Do you suffer from nasal congestion, sneezing, running nose etc?

☐ Do you suffer from rashes, itches, asthma or shortness of breath?

☐ Do you have recurrent colds or sinus problems?

☐ Do you suffer from water retention?

☐ Do you suffer from headaches or migraines?

☐ Do you suffer from other aches or pains from time to time, possibly after certain foods?

☐ Do you suffer from 'brain fog' or patches of inexplicable depression?

☐ Do you get better on holidays abroad, when your diet is completely different?

Any 'yes' answer to these questions means there's a real possibility that you have an allergy. If you score four or more 'yes's', it's pretty much guaranteed.

The telltale signs of food allergy

One of the telltale signs that you might be allergic to something you're eating is that the symptoms come and go. One day you feel fine; the next your joints are aching, or you've got a headache, are blocked up or bloated, and you don't know why. Since most food allergies are delayed (we discuss this in Chapter 2), symptoms often only develop hours after eating the food, making it difficult to put two and two together. (Even more confusing, eating the food you're allergic to can make you feel better immediately afterwards, and only later become problematic.)

Another sign is that you feel better when your diet changes dramatically. For example, if you go on an exotic holiday and eat foods you never usually do, you may, by chance, exclude a food to which you are allergic. (Of course, there are other reasons why you might feel better on holiday: you might be less stressed, for instance.)

Yet many people never vary their menus, and eat the same foods every single day. In our clinics we have seen hundreds of patients whose whole lives have been allergic reactions. For as long as they can remember, they've felt tired or bloated, and suffered from headaches, asthma, eczema or other classic allergic symptoms. And every day of their lives they've eaten wheat or dairy products, say – classic allergens.

It's impossible to know how well you can feel if you've never felt that good. Cathy B is a case in point.

For three years Cathy suffered from joint pain and swelling in her hands, ankles and arms, shooting pains in her arms and legs, unexplained weight gain and fluid retention, extreme fatigue (despite sleeping up to 16 hours a day), uncontrollable food cravings, heartburn, skin rash and heart palpitations despite taking several prescription medications. An IgG food allergy test (see page 85) showed that she was reacting to several foods, including dairy, eggs, sugar cane, yeast, bananas and scallops. She immediately cut all of these foods out of her diet. During the first days off these foods she had a terrible 'killer headache'. Gradually her symptoms began to abate. Within one week she definitely felt better and after seven weeks of following the diet, Cathy was symptom- and medication-free. She had also lost 15lb (nearly 7kg). Once during this time, she broke the diet and the next day many of her symptoms returned, fortunately only temporarily.

Now, let's take a closer look at the two main kinds of food allergies.

2

Immediate and Delayed-onset Food Allergies

IF YOU WERE to lay your small intestine flat on the ground, its surface area would equal that of a small football pitch! This barrier is the gateway between your body and the outside world – your 'inner skin'. Only food substances on the guest list, such as vitamins, minerals, amino acids from digested proteins and so on are allowed through – at least in theory. The police force guarding your inner gateway is your immune system.

■ Food as invader

A food allergy develops when your immune system treats a food you've eaten as an invader, not a friend. This can happen for a number of reasons. In some cases, the food may contain a kind of protein that the body doesn't like. For example, many people's immune system will react to gliadin, a protein abundant in wheat, rye and barley. This can be an inherited condition.

In most cases, food allergies develop when the inside lining of the digestive tract becomes permeable or abnormally 'leaky' because of antibiotic use, excess alcohol consumption, gut infection, excessive physical or emotional stress or other reasons. (We'll discuss these more in Chapter 6 when we show you how to decrease your allergic potential.) The leakiness enables food proteins to 'gatecrash' your bloodstream, and your immune system will react to these outright strangers by attacking them.

This reaction happens on a number of fronts. Your immune system attaches the equivalent of handcuffs to it, called antibodies; attacks and destroys it with specialised cells such as phagocytes; and releases all sorts of reactive chemicals, such as histamine, which also cause many of the symptoms we experience as allergic reactions.

The two most common types of allergic reaction, namely the immediate-onset and the much more common delayed-onset, involve two different families of antibodies, called IgE and IgG respectively. The 'Ig' stands for immunoglobulin, while 'E' or 'G' is the type or family of immunoglobulin. Let's take a closer look at these two different kinds of allergies to see whether or not you are likely to have one.

■ Immediate-onset food allergies (IgE)

The best-known and most studied form of food allergy involves the IgE family of antibodies, and is also known as a Type 1, immediate-onset or atopic food allergy. These allergies are considered 'classic' partly because they were documented in medicine first, and partly because of the immediate and obvious reaction they involve. These are the allergies you read about in the newspaper, when someone dies from eating shellfish or peanuts.

However, immediate-onset allergies are rare: fewer than 5 per cent of us have them, and they are found mostly in children. If you are one of the 2 in 100 adults to have an IgE allergy, you almost certainly know about it because the reactions usually involve only 1 or 2 foods and appear within seconds or up to only 2 hours later. So the condition is usually self-diagnosed and you will already have stopped eating the foods in question.

Immediate-onset allergies can be genetic: you can inherit a tendency to manufacture a specific type of IgE antibody to certain foods. This is why a very serious gluten allergy, coeliac

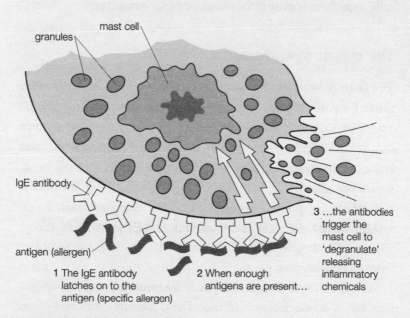

mast cell

granules

IgE antibody

antigen (allergen)

1 The IgE antibody latches on to the antigen (specific allergen)

2 When enough antigens are present...

3 ...the antibodies trigger the mast cell to 'degranulate' releasing inflammatory chemicals

How IgE food allergies happen

disease, runs in families (we discuss coeliac disease in more detail in later chapters, and in Appendix 3, page 156).

Here's how IgE food allergies happen.

One side of the IgE antibody is designed to recognise and tenaciously bind to the food allergen. Before this happens, however, the other side of the IgE antibody must become attached to a troublesome, unstable immune cell called a mast cell. Mast cells are found almost everywhere in the human body, but are especially concentrated in the lining of your digestive tract. Primed for action, the IgE-coated mast cells patiently wait for the allergen to appear.

When you eat that food, the IgE antibodies on the surface of mast cells hungrily latch onto it. Instantaneously, histamine and other allergy-related chemicals come gushing out of the mast cells, rapidly bringing on a range of nasty symptoms.

The classic symptoms

The skin, gut and airways are the usual arena for IgE allergic reactions. So you may see a rash, urticaria (nettle rash) or eczema. You may start to vomit, or experience nausea, stomach cramps, dull aching, bloating, heartburn, indigestion, constipation, flatulence or diarrhoea. (Most people diagnosed with irritable bowel syndrome are found to have food allergies.) Other immediate symptoms include the coughing and wheezing associated with asthma or the sneezing and stuffy nose of a person with allergic rhinitis. The frequency and severity of the reactions vary greatly from person to person.

At the extreme end of the scale, the person can develop anaphylaxis – a reaction where throat and mouth swell and severe asthma comes on, resulting in death from suffocation.

Anaphylactic reactions can also include a kind of nettle rash, rapid dropping of blood pressure, an irregular heartbeat and loss of consciousness.

Here are some of the more common conditions where IgE food allergy may play a part:

- Allergic dermatitis, eczema

- Angioedema (swelling of the skin, for example on the lips)

- Psoriasis

- Asthma

- Interstitial cystitis (recurrent urinary tract infections with no known cause)

- Epilepsy

- Non-seasonal allergic rhinitis (nasal irritation not connected to hay fever, for instance)

- Ulcerative colitis

- Crohn's disease.

On top of identifying and avoiding allergens, there are other ways of reducing your allergic potential, and the amount of histamine released, without resorting to anti-allergic medication. We'll discuss this in Chapter 7.

■ Delayed-onset food allergy (IgG)

IgG allergic reactions are much more common than the IgE type in both children and adults, affecting as many as one in three people – and among those with chronic conditions unresponsive to conventional medicine, up to 70 per cent.

Also known as Type 3 allergies, these occur when your immune system creates an overabundance of IgG antibodies to a particular food allergen. The antibodies, instead of attaching to mast cells like their IgE counterparts, bind directly to the food particles as they enter your bloodstream, creating 'immune complexes'. The more of these you have floating around the bloodstream, the more on edge your immune system becomes, sending out phagocytes to gobble the complexes up. Basically, your immune system gradually goes into red alert.

This process takes time, which is why IgG symptoms are delayed and only appear two hours to several days after consuming the allergen. For example, a migraine headache characteristically appears 48 hours after the allergen is eaten.

These delayed reactions can involve almost any organ or tissue in the human body, potentially provoking over 100 allergic

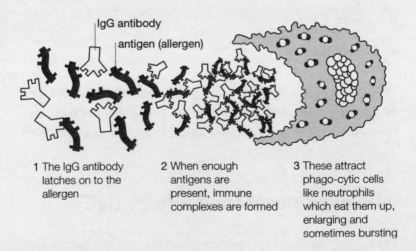

IgG antibody

antigen (allergen)

1 The IgG antibody latches on to the allergen

2 When enough antigens are present, immune complexes are formed

3 These attract phago-cytic cells like neutrophils which eat them up, enlarging and sometimes bursting

How IgG food allergies happen

symptoms and implicated in well over 100 medical diseases and conditions. Here is a partial list of the more common conditions caused or aggravated by IgG food allergy. (We'll be discussing many of these conditions in more detail in the next chapter.)

- Allergic rhinitis, non-seasonal

- Ankylosing spondylitis

- Anxiety, panic attacks

- Asthma (may involve both IgG and IgE antibodies at the same time)

- Attention deficit hyperactivity disorder (ADHD)

- Autism (associated with milk and gluten cereal allergies)

- Bed-wetting

- Depression

- Diabetes, insulin-dependent (gluten, soya and milk casein are primary culprits)

- Eczema (may involve both IgG and IgE antibodies at the same time)

- Epilepsy (with history of migraines or hyperactivity)

- Fatigue, chronic

- Fibromyalgia

- Headaches (migraines, cluster)

- Inflammatory bowel disease (cow's milk enterocolitis, Crohn's disease, ulcerative colitis, and coeliac disease)

- Iron deficiency anaemia

- Irritable bowel syndrome

- Middle ear disease (acute or serous otitis media)

- Rheumatoid arthritis

- Sleep disorders (insomnia, sleep apnoea, snoring).

An estimated one in four people suffer from clinically significant food allergies, most of them from delayed symptoms that are probably the result of IgG food allergies. Unlike IgE allergies, IgG food allergies are very common, and rarely self-diagnosed or treated.

And that's why the main focus of this book is to help you identify any hidden, probably IgG-based, food allergies, as well as how to get rid of or alleviate the symptoms.

■ Understanding the difference between IgE and IgG food allergies

Remember the scene in the movie *Mrs Doubtfire* where Robin Williams, out of blind jealousy, almost kills his ex-wife's allergic suitor with cayenne pepper? That was such an extreme example of an immediate-onset IgE food allergy that the cause-and-effect relationship between food and symptoms was obvious to every viewer.

As we've seen, the symptoms of a delayed-onset IgG food allergy are far more subtle and insidious, and the condition differs in a number of other ways from IgE allergies. We've summed up those differences in the following list:

- Once thought to be the only 'true' food allergy, the immediate-onset type is most common in children, but very rare in adults. Once thought to be uncommon at best, delayed-onset food allergy is by far the most common form of food allergy in children *and* adults.

- Allergic symptoms in immediate reactions occur within two hours of eating. In delayed reactions, symptoms do not appear for at least 2 hours, not infrequently showing up 24 to 48 hours later (and there are even reports of delayed symptoms appearing 3 to 7 days after eating).

- Immediate-onset food allergy involves one or two foods in the diet, as a rule. Delayed reactions characteristically involve 3 to 10 foods, and sometimes as many as 20 foods in very allergic individuals, who are usually found to have highly 'leaky' guts.

- Because a small amount of a single food is involved and the allergic symptoms appear immediately, immediate food allergy is usually self-diagnosed: you eat the food, the symptom swiftly appears, you see the connection and you stop eating it. Due to delayed symptoms, multiple foods and food cravings, delayed-onset food allergies are rarely self-diagnosed, and require the skills of a health professional knowledgeable about food allergies who can run the necessary tests.

- Immediate food allergy involves foods that are rarely eaten. Delayed food allergy involves foods you may well eat every day and even crave.

- When people quit eating foods that cause immediate symptoms, they have no withdrawal or detoxification symptoms, and don't crave or miss these foods. But powerful addictive cravings and disabling withdrawal symptoms are reported in at least one in three people when they stop eating offending IgG foods.

- Immediate reactions to foods primarily affect the skin, airways and digestive tract. Virtually any tissue, organ or system of the body can be affected by delayed food allergy.

- Immediate food allergy can often be diagnosed with a simple skin test. Delayed reactions to food often require state-of-the-art blood tests that detect the presence of specific IgG antibodies to foods in your blood. (We'll be discussing these tests in Chapter 6.)

If you suspect you have an IgE allergy, it's important to get yourself tested and then strictly avoid the substance in question.

Now let's take a look at the most common health problems associated with food allergy.

3

Diseases and Disorders Linked to Food Allergies

WHAT DO WEIGHT gain, eczema and depression have in common? You may be surprised to know that they can all be symptoms of food allergy. If you're eating foods you're allergic to, your digestion, energy levels, sinuses, skin and mental health can all suffer, as Liz's story shows.

case study

Diagnosed with depression at the age of 15, Liz spent the next two years on heavy-duty medication. Then she saw a nutritionist who found she was allergic to wheat. Once she stopped eating it, her depression lifted and she no longer needs anti-depressants. However, if she has any wheat, even inadvertently in a sauce, she becomes depressed, confused, anxious and forgetful for three to four days.

If you have any of these symptoms and they haven't responded to conventional treatment, or get better or worse when you change your diet (for instance, on holiday), then it's

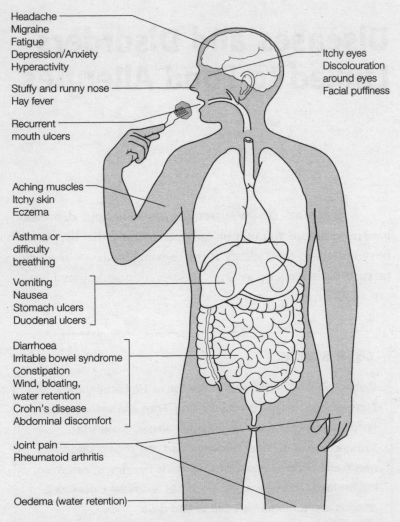

Headache
Migraine
Fatigue
Depression/Anxiety
Hyperactivity

Stuffy and runny nose
Hay fever

Recurrent
mouth ulcers

Itchy eyes
Discolouration
around eyes
Facial puffiness

Aching muscles
Itchy skin
Eczema

Asthma or
difficulty
breathing

Vomiting
Nausea
Stomach ulcers
Duodenal ulcers

Diarrhoea
Irritable bowel syndrome
Constipation
Wind, bloating,
water retention
Crohn's disease
Abdominal discomfort

Joint pain
Rheumatoid arthritis

Oedema (water retention)

Symptoms associated with food allergy

well worth investigating whether a hidden food allergy is involved.

■ Inflammatory bowel diseases and IBS

Since food allergies are triggered by immune reactions in the gut, or by a leaky gut (see page 100) that allows incompletely digested proteins from food to enter the bloodstream, it is hardly surprising that many digestive symptoms are linked to food allergy.

Inflammatory bowel diseases

When a person bloats after eating, or experiences abdominal pain, constipation and/or diarrhoea and excessive flatulence, the first medical prerogative is to find out whether inflammation, bleeding or ulceration is involved.

There are three common types of inflammatory bowel disease: Crohn's disease, ulcerative colitis and coeliac disease. Common symptoms for all three are pain in the joints, lack of appetite, weight loss and fever.

In Crohn's disease, the wall of the intestine becomes sore, inflamed, and swollen. In ulcerative colitis, tiny sores form in the inner lining of the colon and rectum. In addition to the symptoms mentioned above, both of these conditions are characterised by abdominal pain and cramps, diarrhoea, rectal bleeding and/or bloody stools. There are no lab tests to help identify either disease, and diagnosis is usually based on a medical history, a physical examination and X-rays. Conventional treatment for both involves minor adjustments to the diet (for example, a decrease in fat, fibre and lactose), anti-inflammatory drugs and sometimes antibiotics for local infections.

Coeliac disease is more than twice as common in the general population as Crohn's, ulcerative colitis and cystic fibrosis combined. There are often no abdominal symptoms in the early stages. Unlike Crohn's and ulcerative colitis, coeliac disease can be diagnosed with sophisticated lab tests and intestinal biopsies of the lining of the small intestine (more on this later). The only effective treatment is total and life-time elimination of gluten grains from the diet, which means no wheat (including variants and hybrids such as kamut, triticale and spelt), rye or barley. Oats may need to be cut out, too, although many people with coeliac disease can tolerate them.

If you have inflammatory bowel disease, there's a very good chance you've got a food allergy. One study of patients with colitis found that sufferers were ten times more likely to have an IgG allergy to eggs or soya.[5] In another study, people with ulcerative colitis were more likely to react to gliadin, a protein found in gluten in wheat, rye and barley (but not oats). Crohn's sufferers were also more likely to react to yeast.[6] In truth, everyone is different and it's well worth having a IgG allergy test if you have either of these conditions.

Irritable bowel syndrome (IBS)

If you have symptoms of bloating, abdominal pain, flatulence and intermittent constipation and/or diarrhoea but there's no evidence of inflammation, then you'll probably be diagnosed as having irritable bowel syndrome, or IBS. The most common symptom is a crampy, colicky pain or a continuous dull aching in the lower abdomen, often relieved after passing gas or having a bowel movement.

This debilitating condition wasn't really taken seriously until recently. This is illustrated by the story of Denise Lewis, one of Britain's best-known athletes, who won a gold medal for the heptathlon at the Sydney Olympics in 2000 and starred in the hit TV show *Strictly Come Dancing*. What no one knew was that for the past 13 years she has suffered from Irritable Bowel Syndrome.

case study

For 13 years I've suffered from an excruciating and incurable stomach disorder called Irritable Bowel Syndrome (IBS). At times it's left me curled up in agony, feeling as if someone was wringing out my guts by hand, and there is nothing I can do – not standing, sitting or lying down – that can make the pain go away. Suddenly, I'll get a desperate urge to go to the loo and only then do I feel any relief.

I first started getting the symptoms of IBS in 1992 – bloating, constipation and wind, followed by terrible stomach pains. Like most sufferers, I wrote off the attacks as isolated incidents because they occurred months apart.

Then, in the summer of 1993, at an athletics competition in Birmingham, I had a particularly bad attack. It was the morning of my javelin event and the attack lasted more than two hours. I spent the run-up to the event trying every which way to get comfortable and praying for it to be over. Finally, the pain went, and somehow I managed to get out there and win. After that attack I went to my GP, who referred me to a gastric specialist. He carried out an endoscopy. When the ▶

specialist didn't find anything, I was sent away with some anti-acid pills and Fybrogel, a medicine to help with my constipation. They didn't really help. In essence, I was told that I just had to learn to live with it.

I started keeping a food diary to see if anything I was eating was triggering the attacks, but there seemed to be no real pattern. Then I looked at my menstrual cycle; but again there was no link.

I cut out coffee and rich foods, including my favourite ice cream, but if anything the attacks seemed more frequent. By 1998, I was having around one attack a month. Finally, in 1998, after an attack during which I vomited, I knew it was time to look for help again.

This time, I was referred to a private clinic in London's Devonshire Place, where I had an endoscopy and a colonoscopy, The doctor could see some irritation, but, overall, my stomach, intestines and bowels were pretty healthy. While he couldn't see a reason for the spasms, he was the first person to give my problem a name – Irritable Bowel Syndrome, which was a disorder of not just the bowel but the entire intestines. He said it could be stress related, but the truth was that no one really knew why IBS occurred. I was prescribed Fybogel again but it didn't really make any difference. At that time, I had no option but to learn to live with it. It was the run-up to the Sydney Olympics and I didn't have time to worry about being ill or in pain. I had attacks every couple of months, mostly at home in the evenings, but I just had to sweat through it and carry on with my rigorous training routine.

▶

Then, in October last year, I heard about blood tests that could be done to establish if you were suffering from food allergies. I'd never really considered it before, because my own food diary had proved so inconclusive, but now I felt I had nothing to lose. All I had to do was prick my finger with a pin, let the blood collect in a special container and then send off the sample.

About a week later, I received the results of the tests. The report said I was very intolerant of cow's milk, moderately intolerant of yeast and egg white, and mildly intolerant of egg yolk, garlic and cashew nuts. I wasn't surprised about the cow's milk. I regularly felt uncomfortable after drinking it, and had often drunk soya milk and eaten dairy-free products.

Since removing these foods almost a year ago I haven't had a single attack. It's not always easy to avoid the foods but the benefits are worth it for a pain-free existence. Finding out what I'm allergic to with the IgG allergy test has transformed my life. For the first time in 13 years I'm pain free.

Next to the common cold, IBS symptoms are the most commonly reported ailment, affecting as many as one in four people. It is most likely to appear in late teens and early adulthood and is four times more common in women than men. IBS sufferers often have a history of antibiotic use, which might increase the risk of developing food allergies.

If diagnosed, you might be given bran supplements, but these are rarely effective[7] and can sometimes make matters worse.[8] It's far more effective to find out which foods you're specifically allergic to, and eliminate them.

To test this approach, researchers at the University of York in the UK devised an ingenious study.[9] They tested 150 IBS sufferers using an IgG allergy test and then gave their doctors either real or fake results, and a supposedly 'allergy-free' diet to follow for the next three months. Neither the patients nor their doctors knew that some of the diagnoses – and thus, the diets – were fake.

At the end of the three-month trial there was a significant improvement only in those who'd been following a diet that cut out foods they were actually allergic to. What's more, those who stuck to it most strictly had the best results. Other studies have also shown that IBS sufferers have a higher incidence of IgG allergies than non-sufferers.[10] And as IgE allergies are not so common in IBS sufferers, it is important to test for any hidden IgG allergies.

Sandra didn't have coeliac disease, but she was gluten sensitive, as many people with IBS are.[11–13] Some are lactose intolerant. Either way, the best thing to do is to have an IgG allergy test.

■ Weight gain and water retention

If you're carrying excess weight, chances are it could be partly due to allergy. Rebecca's story shows how it can happen.

case study

In her twenties, Rebecca's weight was stable and her skin good. She used to exercise three or four times a week. But in her thirties she started to pile on the pounds. Over three years her weight drifted from 140lb (64kg) to over 180lb (80kg), ▶

and her dress size went up to 16. She also developed itchy patches on her face and had a lot of colds and sinus trouble. She didn't exercise because she didn't feel good. 'I started feeling tired and lethargic and generally unwell,' she said. 'I didn't have the energy to go to the gym any more.'

For breakfast she'd have toast, then a main meal of meat and potatoes with gravy for lunch, and a sandwich for dinner. 'But it seemed like the foods I ate were blowing me up, which is why I thought I could have a food allergy.' She decided to test herself for a food allergy using a home test kit. The results showed she was reacting to milk, egg white and gluten (in wheat, barley and rye). Within a week of excluding these foods she found that her skin and mood improved and the weight started to fall away without her consciously restricting calories. After six months she had lost 42lb (19kg).

After three months of strictly avoiding the foods she'd become allergic to, she reintroduced egg whites and then milk to see if there was a reaction. Now she's fine on both foods, but still reacts to wheat.

'I can't tell you how much better I feel. I'm 100 per cent,' she said. 'It has transformed my health. Having the food intolerance test has been the best thing I've done. I wish I'd done it sooner.' In the end, she shed all the weight she'd gained during the previous three years.

Rebecca's dramatic weight gain – and loss – was unlikely to have been down solely to fat. Food allergies can cause oedema, or water retention, which can also pile on the pounds. You might be holding as much as 10lb (4.5kg) of extra fluid or even more without realising it. In fact, you can easily gain up to 14lb in body weight this way – and lose all that in as little as 48 hours if you eliminate the allergen.

---

case study

Marie was a case in point. She is allergic to wheat but insisted on eating it while on vacation in Hawaii. Her fingers swelled so much and so quickly that her marriage ring began cutting into her finger, causing bleeding. She had to have the ring cut off in an emergency room as a consequence.

How can you tell whether your weight gain is mainly fat, or substantially due to oedema? Just answer this questionnaire.

Are you waterlogged?

☐ Do you ever experience sudden fluctuations in your weight?

☐ Do you easily gain – and then lose – 3 to 5lb (1.5 to 2.3kg) or more in a day?

☐ Does your face look puffy, especially around and under the eyes?

☐ Do you have noticeable bags under your eyes?

☐ Does your abdomen, on pressing, feel waterlogged and bloated?

Do you have to loosen your belt after eating?

Do your arms feel puffy rather than like pure fat and muscle?

Do both of your ankles ever swell up?

Do your fingers ever swell up so it's hard to get your rings off?

Do you have dry skin or dandruff?

Do you suffer from breast tenderness?

Are you prone to allergies?

If you answer 'yes' to three or more of the questions above, chances are that water retention is partly – or mainly – to blame for your weight problem.

But a food allergy isn't the only reason for water retention. Blood sugar problems, kidney problems, sodium excess and essential fat deficiency can also promote watery weight gain. Here's what you can do to rule these out:

- Avoid sugary or refined foods and stimulants such as coffee

- Eat five servings of a variety of fruits and vegetables every day

- Eat seeds (rich in essential fats, plus magnesium and potassium)

- Eat wholefoods and wholegrains such as beans, lentils, brown rice and wholegrain bread (be aware that you may be

gluten sensitive and have to avoid wholewheat, rye and
barley)

- Eat more oily fish such as mackerel (rich in essential fats) in
  unfried and unbreaded form, and less meat

- Don't add salt to your food, unless it's low-sodium salt such
  as Solo salt

- Choose 'low sodium' processed foods

- Drink the equivalent of eight glasses of water, including
  herbal teas, a day.

This way of eating alone may cause you to rapidly lose weight if
water retention is part of your problem. But if you are finding it
hard to shift weight, the most important thing is to find out
which foods you are allergic to and stay off them.

Weight and waterlogging: how it happens

How do food allergies lead to waterlogging? First, histamine,
the stuff that makes you sneeze when it's in your nose,
makes tiny blood vessels called capillaries leakier. This
allows the immune system's army of white blood cells to
move into the battlefield – your tissues. At the same time,
fluid accompanying the white blood cells passes into your
tissues, where it's retained for days, even weeks. If this is
happening several times a day, you literally become waterlogged.

   Allergic reactions also mess up the balance of
prostaglandins, hormone-like substances made from ▶

essential fats, and this too can lead to water retention as well as abdominal bloating.

Take the case of Joanne M. She didn't just have weight to lose, but girth.

But there's more to the weight gain than water. The more frequent your allergic reactions, the more resistant you become to insulin, the hormone that keeps your blood sugar in balance. This is because the body releases masses of immune messengers called cytokines to deal with the allergy, and cytokines make you less responsive to insulin. Also, repeated allergic reactions mean that more garbage – that is, immune complexes – ends up in your bloodstream as your immune cells struggle, often unsuccessfully, to fight off the invaders.

It's up to your liver, your body's detoxifying organ, to clean up the ensuing mess. But eventually, your liver's detox capacity will get overloaded. When this happens, your body dumps the toxins in the least harmful place – your fat cells. The more intoxicated your fat cells become, the slower the body's ability to metabolise fat, and the more fat is retained; and the more weight you gain, the harder it becomes to shift those extra pounds. This is why people with allergies can find it harder and harder to lose weight. Also, this continual process of over-intoxication can turn a mild food allergy into something more severe. It also invariably leads to chronic fatigue.

case study

I used to stand in front of the mirror, grab a handful of my tummy – and despair. After a big meal I looked five months pregnant! It wasn't just my weight, which hovered around 154lb (70kg), it was the bloating (I'd gone up to a size 16) and the physical symptoms. I'd have to undo my trousers every time I had a big meal and I was often constipated.

When I was in my late teens, I was diagnosed with IBS. Instead of looking for the cause, doctors simply prescribed drugs to ease the symptoms. Reading up about the problem, I got the impression a high-fibre diet would help the constipation and stop my tummy from bloating. But my health regime of wholemeal bread, baked potatoes and beans was actually making it worse.

I felt exhausted all the time and usually fell asleep by 9.30 in the evening. My husband Steve kept telling me I had to do something about it. So in September 2002 I sent away for a food intolerance blood test. The results told me I was sensitive to all dairy products, yeast, salmon, trout, haricot beans and string beans. Within a week I was going to the loo every two days (instead of weekly), my tummy was gone and I was down to a size 12. My lethargy was caused by the yeasty foods I ate. I've gone down to 129lb (59kg) and look so much trimmer now.

▪ Fatigue and insomnia

Fatigue is the reason for so many doctors' visits that a new term has been coined – TATT ('tired all the time'). More than half of people diagnosed with chronic fatigue syndrome (CFS) also have allergies to foods, airborne substances and drugs, according to one scientific review.[14] Another study reports that about 50 per cent of CFS patients have 'non-allergic rhinitis', meaning they have nasal symptoms that are unrelated to an IgE allergy.[15] Most likely, in our opinion, these symptoms are caused or aggravated by IgG food allergies.

If you're having trouble getting a good night's sleep, food allergy might be contributing. Food allergies are certainly not the only reasons for fatigue and insomnia but if you are tired all the time or unable to sleep or both, and haven't been able to identify a cause, then getting tested for a food allergy is a sensible route to follow.

■ Headaches and migraines

Frequent headaches or migraines are extremely debilitating. One migraine sufferer put it this way: 'When I had headaches, I only lived half a life. When I had a migraine, everything else was obliterated by the pain – my family, my work, my name. I was living half my life on another planet, a planet of torture and pain.'

Migraines are thought to happen when arteries in the scalp dilate, and those in the brain constrict. Aside from the pain, they may involve visual disturbances, nausea, vomiting and sensitivity to light and noise. It's an exhausting experience, and the sufferer usually has to sleep it off afterwards. They affect more women than men, and about one in ten people.

A cluster headache is the most severe of all headaches, found more often in men than women. It often comes on during sleep and/or 20 to 40 minutes after drinking alcohol. Sufferers will experience severe pain, usually behind one eye, described as feeling like a red-hot poker being driven into the eye socket. They can last for hours or even days non-stop, often occur in batches on a daily basis, and can also bring on symptoms such as tearing in the affected eye; a stuffed-up nose; feeling hot; a sweaty face, neck and trunk; nausea, vomiting and/or diarrhoea; a drop in blood pressure; and even heart arrhythmia. Unsurprisingly, they're incapacitating and can drive sufferers to the brink of their endurance.

While the trigger of both migraines and cluster headaches is still largely unknown, there is growing evidence that in many cases food allergy is the culprit. About a quarter of migraine patients report that their symptoms can be initiated by certain foods.[16] One double-blind study on 40 children with migraines reported a decrease of attacks in over 80 per cent of children who avoided some foods. Associated symptoms also improved, including abdominal pain, fits, asthma and eczema.[17] Other studies have observed a decrease in the number of attacks in 80 per cent of patients on avoidance diets.[18-19] We believe that testing and eliminating food allergens should be the first avenue of attack on migraine and cluster headaches, not the last.

case study

Alison suffered increasingly severe headaches and migraines for ten years. Often the headaches would be accompanied by sickness and flashing lights, and she would have to retreat into a darkened room to rest for a day and two nights. She also suffered from a 'fuzzy' head and felt very lethargic.

Since doctors could not offer a solution other than painkillers to help ease the pain, she had an IgG food ▶

allergy test. The results showed an intolerance to dairy products, yeast, seafood and nuts.

Within a couple of days of cutting these foods out of her diet, she began to feel better. Her head felt clearer, her energy levels improved and her symptoms of sinusitis and rheumatoid arthritis also eased considerably. The number of migraines she had dropped dramatically. Recently, she ate half a cheese sandwich – and rediscovered the importance of sticking to her avoidance diet. 'By the end of the afternoon, I could feel a headache coming on,' she said. 'It was bad the next day and only eased off the day after that.'

In our experience, the majority of migraine and cluster headaches can be traced to delayed-onset food allergy. The most common allergic villains in migraines and headaches (and there's often more than one) are cow's milk, eggs, wheat, oranges, benzoic acid, cheese, rye, tomato and chemical additives, especially tartrazine and MSG. Typically, the time lag between eating an offending food and developing a headache or migraine is 48 hours, which makes it harder to self-diagnose. As the food allergy implicated in migraines is almost always delayed-onset, we recommend an IgG allergy test.

■ Arthritis and joint pain

Arthritis is a debilitating disease that affects 9 out of 10 people by the age of 60. There are two kinds – osteoarthritis and rheumatoid arthritis. The most common is osteoarthritis, affecting joints that have been injured or simply worn out, often through poor posture and lack of mobility, which is necessary to keep joints flexible and healthy. It usually comes on after 50.

Rheumatoid arthritis, however, can strike at any age and affects about 1 in 100 people, mostly women. This is an inflammatory disease that causes pain, swelling, stiffness, and loss of function in the joints, and can also affect other parts of the body. It is also an autoimmune condition: there is evidence that the body's own immune system attacks the joints. People with the disease may experience fatigue, occasional fever and a general sense of malaise. It can be mild, or severe and active most of the time, last for many years, and lead to serious joint damage and disability. It is so disabling that half of patients have to stop working within ten years of diagnosis.

No conventional treatment can cure or reverse rheumatoid arthritis, but there are medications that can relieve its symptoms and slow or halt its progress. They include non-steroidal anti-inflammatory drugs (to help relieve pain and inflammation), corticosteroids (to reduce inflammation and slow joint damage) and disease-modifying anti-rheumatic drugs (to slow or halt the progression of rheumatoid arthritis). Each of these treatments has side effects – stomach upset/bleeding, easy bruising, thinning of bones, cataracts, weight gain, diabetes, high blood pressure, blurry vision and increased susceptibility to infection. There is also recent evidence that after about ten years on these medications, the degeneration of the joint tissue begins to accelerate, while surgical joint replacement seems to encourage more joint instability.

With rheumatoid arthritis, as with other autoimmune diseases like lupus or Type 1 diabetes, it's well worth suspecting food allergy as the trigger – especially gluten, soya and/or dairy sensitivities. Our 25 years of clinical experience have taught us that rheumatoid arthritis is frequently caused or provoked by food allergy, and that most rheumatoid arthritics under the age of 70 respond dramatically to food allergy elimination, together with an optimum nutrition diet and supplements, including natural anti-inflammatory nutrients and herbs such as omega-3 fish oil, curcumin, boswellia and hop extracts, to name a few. (See Patrick's book *Say No to Arthritis* for a comprehensive nutrition-based strategy.)

One theory about why food allergy could trigger autoimmune conditions is that the immune system could become sensitive to a food protein such as soya or milk protein, and wrongly 'cross-react' to tissue in the body (which is, of course, largely protein). While an allergy-free diet doesn't help everybody, studies do show that some people experience great benefits. In one, 9 per cent of a group of rheumatoid arthritis patients improved when put on an allergy-free diet, and worsened when taken off it. To make sure these results were real, six of these patients were reintroduced to small amounts of non-allergic foods or allergic foods without their knowing which they were taking. Four got noticeably worse on the allergy food, not the placebo.[20]

case study

John developed both psoriasis and arthritis in his toes, fingers, ankles and knees at the age of 23. By 40 he couldn't sleep at night from the pain and had to go upstairs on hands and knees. Walking just 100 yards was painful. Holidays were awful. He used to have to think carefully where to park the car

▶

when going out so as not to have to walk too far. He saw consultants, read books and took lots of medication, which controlled the pain but had their own side effects – stomach pain and depression. Sometimes he had steroid injections to make the pain subside, but it would return later in the day.

Then John heard about food allergy testing. Although his GP actively discouraged testing of that type, saying that there was 'absolutely no clinical evidence' that altering diet would improve such a condition, John went ahead and discovered he was allergic to three different foods. He was shocked to discover that the main one was white fish, as everyone had been saying to cut out red meat and eat much more white and oily fish. Egg white was another – and the last was tea. John cut them all out. Gradually the number of painkillers he needed lessened and eventually he stopped completely. In his own words, 'Life is now pain- and tablet-free and I have complete mobility. I am amazed at the difference in my quality of life simply by making such simple adjustments.'

While food allergy isn't the only factor contributing to arthritis, we recommend exploring it if you do suffer from arthritis or joint aches and pains.

■ Eczema and other skin problems

Eczema can vary from mild to severe. In mild forms the skin is dry, hot and itchy, while in more severe forms the skin can become broken, raw and bleeding. Conventional treatment involves anti-inflammatory skin creams – usually betnovate, a form of cortisone. This reduces the severity but the skin remains sensitive to flare-ups.

The causes of eczema are many and varied, and depend on the particular type a person has. Atopic eczema is thought to be a hereditary condition, and is diagnosed if the affected person has other allergic symptoms and/or a family history of such conditions, including asthma and hay fever. It is highly likely that a person with this form of eczema has food and possibly chemical and/or inhalant allergies. Other types of eczema are caused by irritants such as chemicals and detergents, allergens such as nickel, and yeast growths. In later years eczema can be caused by a circulatory problem in the legs. The causes of other types of eczema remain to be explained, though links with environmental factors and stress are being explored.

The most common food allergy that can provoke eczema, especially in children, is milk. IgG antibodies to milk have been found to be much more common in both children and adults with eczema.[21-25] Other investigators have also found IgG sensitivity to eggs to be far more common in eczema sufferers.[26] Despite overwhelming evidence of an association with hidden IgG food allergy, very few eczema sufferers are tested for allergy by their doctors.

case study

Liza is a case in point. She had suffered from eczema, and had used betnovate and other steroid-based creams, all her life. Her eczema was worst on her hands and arms. She has

▶

been to a herbalist who charged her hundreds of pounds to carry out so-called allergy tests. He used an electronic machine 'that looked like it was out of the 1950s', placing it on the palm of her hand and then listening to the beeps the machine made. He claimed that the noises determined her food sensitivities. He told her to cut out a long list of foods and also recommended that she take 13 tablets a day.

Liza did manage to stick to the diet – and her eczema got so bad that her skin blistered. After four days her eczema was worse than ever and it took another two and a half weeks for it to improve at all. Not surprisingly, she didn't stick with the diet for long.

We tested her using a proper IgG food allergy blood test and found she was strongly allergic to dairy products and mildly sensitive to gluten and egg white. She was also given a vitamin A-based skin cream called Environ Pro-Active. This can help to keep the skin healthy once the inflammation calms down.

In her case, stress made her skin worse and, noticing that she often had several cups of coffee and a couple of Red Bull drinks each day, we recommended she cut out any source of caffeine. (Both stress and caffeine raise levels of the hormones adrenalin and cortisol, leading to increased inflammation.)

One month later this is what she said: 'I feel so much better. Nothing like as tired. I have one coffee a week, no headaches, no side effects. No bloating. The milk avoidance itself wasn't so difficult. But I was amazed to find out how many foods had hidden milk so it took a week to discover what I could and couldn't have. Overall, it's been fine. It's not as hard as it used

►

to be at the beginning. My skin is a lot better. I have no sores and no cuts – it's just a little dry. The vitamin A cream really works very well. I have lost a couple of pounds. I am really surprised how easy I found it to cut out the caffeine, and I have more energy, not less.'

Three months later Liza is still eczema-free and has not had to use the betnovate cream once since she went on her allergy-free diet.

While food allergy is clearly not the only cause of skin problems such as eczema, we believe anyone with eczema, and also conditions like hives and dermatitis, should strongly consider having an IgG food allergy test. In more cases than not, an allergy-free diet makes a big difference.

■ Asthma and nasal and sinus problems

Some of the most common food allergy symptoms are constant coughing, sniffling and snuffling, excessive mucus formation and a blocked nose. This can lead to or be associated with a variety of diseases of the airways, such as asthma, bronchitis, rhinitis (hay fever), and sinusitis. The most serious and life-threatening of these is undoubtedly asthma.

There are more than 5 million asthma sufferers in Britain. That's close to 1 in 12 people! Even with earlier diagnosis and more hospitalisation, deaths from asthma have tripled and the number of new cases diagnosed each year has increased by 160 per cent since 1980. The fatality rate is highest in the elderly and children (see Chapter 4 for a discussion of childhood asthma).

Asthma is primarily an allergic condition because allergens stimulate the release of histamine and leukotrienes, chemical mediators, from sensitised immune cells lining the airways. This causes the airway tubes to become highly irritated. When this happens the tissue in the tubes becomes swollen, and gelatin-like mucus begins to plug up the air passages.

The result is potentially serious bouts of wheezing, and coughing (easily provoked by laughing, exercising, crying or breathing cold air). This may lead on to other symptoms – shortness of breath, pressure in the chest, and difficult breathing or 'tight throat' – which can make asthmatics feel as if they are slowly suffocating to death. An attack may last for a few hours or go on for weeks, and may never get past the wheezing and coughing stage, or may require all a sufferer's energy to keep breathing.

Why is this debilitating disorder becoming more widespread and dangerous? The reasons are many: the declining quality of our diets, stressful or inactive lifestyles, increasing exposure to airborne and food allergens, increased incidence of other allergic conditions (otitis, sinusitis, eczema and a family history of atopic allergies occur more frequently in asthmatics), chemicals and toxins in our environment, overuse of aspirin and aspirin substitutes, sulphites in white wine as well as dried fruits and other processed foods, and an overdependence on inhalers.

In mainstream medicine until recently, the assumption dictating therapy was that asthma was basically an airway-narrowing disease. Consequently, medication to dilate or enlarge the airways is the norm, and so-called inhaled corticosteroids have also been thrown into the mix.

The problems with this approach are threefold: when used excessively (more than a canister and a half per month), inhalers are associated with a dramatic increase in death rates. Long-term use of inhaled corticosteroids don't seem to change the progression of the disease, merely control symptoms, and has other adverse effects in children. What's more, the conventional wisdom that inhalers should be used regularly has been overturned by research that shows you are better off using them as and when you need them (and as little as possible) than having this constant intake of steroids.[27]

A better and more lasting approach to treating asthma – and many nasal or sinus problems – is to address the underlying causes of airway inflammation and hyper-irritability, not just the short-term relief of wheezing, coughing and shortness of breath. This begins with the identification and elimination of airborne and food allergens. The top suspects are wheat, milk and eggs,[28] while colourings, preservatives (especially sulphites) and other chemical food additives may also be implicated, along with dust mites, mould, animal dander and cockroach antigens (proteins from the insects' saliva, eggs and so on).

As you'll see in Chapter 6, improving nutrition will strengthen the immune system and reduce allergic reactions. Also, there are many excellent natural anti-inflammatory herbs and nutrients that can make an asthmatic less dependent on inhalers. Among these are quercitin (see page 125) and butterbur. A recent trial by the University of Heidelberg in Germany, involving 80 adults and children suffering from asthma, found that 40 per cent could reduce their use of medication by taking a daily supplement of butterbur root.[29]

▪ Low moods, 'brain fogs' and depression

Most people don't think of food allergies as a potential cause of low mood, poor concentration, anxiety or even more severe conditions such as schizophrenia. Yet the knowledge that allergy to foods and chemicals can adversely affect moods and behaviour in susceptible individuals has been known for a very long time. Food allergies have been proven to cause a diverse range of symptoms including chronic fatigue, slowed thought processes, lack of motivation, irritability, agitation, aggressive behaviour, nervousness, anxiety, depression, alcoholism and substance abuse, schizophrenia, hyperactivity (ADHD), panic attacks, autism and varied learning disabilities.[30-39]

We'll discuss the link to problems in children in detail in the next chapter.

A doctor from Munich, Joseph Egger, was one of the first pioneers studying the link between allergy and mental health. He decided to test 30 patients suffering from anxiety, depression, confusion or difficulty in concentrating for allergy, using a double-blind placebo-controlled trial, by giving the patients either dummy foods, or their allergenic foods, in small quantities, disguised so they didn't know what they were eating. The results showed that the food allergens alone were able to produce severe depression, nervousness, feeling of anger without a particular object, loss of motivation and severe mental blankness. The foods which produced most severe mental reactions were wheat, milk, cane sugar and eggs.[40]

Another pioneer of food and chemical sensitivity was Dr Benjamin Feingold, whose Feingold Diet became famous in the 1970s. He investigated the possibility of food allergies and sensitivity to salicylates (such as aspirin) in 96 patients diagnosed as suffering from alcohol dependence, major depressive disorders and schizophrenia compared to 62 control subjects selected from adult hospital staff members for a possible food/chemical intolerance.

The results showed that the group of patients diagnosed as depressives had the highest number of allergies: 80 per cent were allergic to barley, and all were allergic to egg white. Over half the alcoholics tested were found to be allergic to egg white, milk, rye and barley. Of the people with schizophrenia, 80 per cent were found to be allergic to both milk and eggs. Only 9 per cent of the control group were found to suffer from any allergies.[41]

These studies are prime examples of how problems created by allergies can often produce a multitude of mental as well as physical symptoms, because they affect the central nervous system, and even the whole body. The state of inflammation induced by an allergic reaction is found in many mental health conditions, from depression to autism, and is probably one of the main mechanisms by which a food allergy affects the brain. What's more, allergies are very specific to the individual, as are the symptoms they create, so any diagnosis can only be made individually by proper food allergy testing.

At the Brain Bio Centre in London we routinely test individuals with mental health issues for allergy. It is not at all uncommon for us to find that putting a person on the allergy-free diet they need relieves symptoms of depression, insomnia, anxiety and even schizophrenia. So if you suffer from poor concentration, insomnia, anxiety or other symptoms of depleted mental health, it's well worth investigating whether food allergies play a part. If you'd like to explore the optimum nutrition approach in its entirety, your best option is to come to the Brain Bio Centre in London (see Resources, page 170).

4

Children and Food Allergies

OF ALL PEOPLE, children show most clearly that our 21st-century diets and lifestyles are resulting in more and more food allergies and sensitivities. And along with those allergies go a wide range of childhood illnesses and other conditions – from middle ear disease to attention deficit hyperactive disorder (ADHD). Let's look at these now.

■ The ADHD epidemic

ADHD is fast becoming a household name. In Britain it is vastly underdiagnosed, yet the symptoms are estimated to occur in a quarter of a million children under the age of 17. In the US the figure is rapidly approaching 3 million.

ADHD affects five times as many boys as girls. A third or more ADHD children will grow up to be ADHD adults. There is no laboratory or clinical test available yet that definitively diagnoses the condition; a diagnosis is based on observations of inattention, hyperactivity and impulsivity so serious they impair a child's ability to function. Many children with ADHD take medication under a doctor's prescription, usually the amphetamine-like drug Ritalin (methylphenidate) to help them pay attention, calm down, become less disruptive and perform better in school. More than 250,000 prescriptions for Ritalin are written each year.

Largely ignored, however, is the role that food allergy and chemical food additive sensitivities play in children with ADHD. In a classic study by Dr Joseph Egger and colleagues at the University of Munich in Germany, 76 children with severe ADHD were kept on a strict hypoallergenic (very low allergic potential) diet for 4 weeks.[42] The results were amazing: 82 per cent of the children got better on the hypoallergenic diet. One out of four children with severe ADHD recovered completely. Even more remarkably, most of the other non-ADHD symptoms improved with the diet, as well. Here's what happened.

Symptom	Number of Children Suffering from It	
	Before diet change	On diet
Antisocial behaviour	32	13
Headaches	48	9
Seizures/fits	14	1
Abdominal pain or discomfort	54	8
Chronic rhinitis	33	9
Leg aches	33	6
Skin rashes	28	9
Mouth ulcers	15	5
Emotional problems	7	0

Egger then gave the children foods with artificial food colours and preservatives. He found the most problematic common substances were the chemical additives tartrazine and benzoic acid (E102 and E210). However, no child reacted to these two food additives alone. A total of 46 different foods provoked allergic symptoms. Soya, cow's milk, wheat, grapes, chocolate, oranges, eggs and peanuts were the most common food allergens. Foods that did not cause symptoms included cabbage, lettuces, cauliflower, celery – and duck eggs!

Having identified which foods each child was allergic to, he then ran a test, giving the children either a placebo or a tiny amount of the food allergen without either the child or the researcher knowing which was given (in other words, a placebo-controlled double-blind test). This showed these children definitely were reacting to specific foods and chemicals.

In the UK, the leading child psychiatrist Professor Eric Taylor was somewhat sceptical about the reports he was getting from parents saying their children were behaving better on diets excluding chemical additives and/or common food allergens. He decided to investigate with another double-blind trial.[43] He took 78 hyperactive children and placed them on a 'few foods' elimination diet. Fifty-nine of the children showed improved behaviour during the trial. For 19 of these children it was possible to disguise foods or additives, or both, that reliably provoked behavioural problems by mixing them with other tolerated foods and to test their effect in a placebo-controlled double-blind design. The results of this trial on these 19 children showed that the provoking foods did worsen ratings of behaviour and impair psychological test performance.

Carrie's story shows how dramatic the improvement can be.

case study

From the age of two, Carrie had suffered from extreme hyper-activity, chronic insomnia, irritability, headaches, frequent sinus and middle ear infections and joint pains, and had dark circles under her eyes. None of the treatments and tests that she underwent brought her any relief. When Carrie was five, her parents had her tested for IgG food allergy. They found their daughter was allergic to 22 different foods. She was also found to have a number of airborne allergies – to mould, house-dust mites, pollens and dog dander. Taking all 22 foods out of her diet and removing some of the sources of airborne allergens from her home improved her symptoms very quickly. At ten, Carrie is very well, with none of her previous symptoms.

■ Autism

Among autistic children the evidence for food allergy, especially allergy to gluten grains and milk, is even higher than for children with ADHD. Much of the impetus for recognising the importance of dietary intervention has come from parents who have noticed vast improvements in their autistic children after changing their diets.

Wheat and dairy products – and the proteins they contain, gluten and casein – are the foods linked most strongly to autism. These proteins are difficult to digest and, especially if introduced too early in life, may result in an allergy. Fragments of them, known as peptides, can mimic chemicals in the brain called endorphins, so they're often referred to as 'exorphins'.

By mimicking the body's own endorphins, which is what heroin does, the body becomes less sensitive to its own natural endorphins, which leads to cravings for even more of these exorphins found in milk and wheat.[44]

The most common food allergies and chemical intolerances in autistic children are:

- Wheat and other gluten-containing grains

- Milk and other dairy products containing casein

- Citrus fruits

- Chocolate

- Salicylates (as in aspirin)

- Foods in the nightshade family (potatoes, tomatoes, aubergines, peppers)

- Paracetamol

- Tartrazine (E102), benzoic acid (E210) and monosodium glutamate (MSG/E621).

If you have a child with autism or Asperger's syndrome, we strongly recommend you investigate food allergy as a contributory cause. If you'd like to find out more about the nutritional approach to autism, see *Optimum Nutrition for the Mind* (Piatkus).

■ Ear, nose and throat infections

Almost every parent is aware of the agony their child experiences with ear infection, which can often involve the nose and throat as well. The most common and serious is middle ear infection, of which there are two types: acute otitis media, and otitis media with effusion (also called serous otitis media, and nick-named 'glue ear'), which involves fluid build-up in the middle ear.

Signs and symptoms of acute otitis media include:

- Severe and persistent pain in one or both ears

- Ear tugging or pulling

- Fever up to 104°F (fever with chills or fever with a headache may be a sign of more serious complications)

- Irritability, lethargy

- Loss of appetite, nausea, vomiting and/or diarrhoea, and concurrent signs of allergic rhinitis (frequent sneezing, runny or congested nose, nose rubbing, eye burning), catarrh and recurrent tonsillitis may also appear in as many as 80 per cent of otitis media sufferers.

In otitis media with effusion, the signs and symptoms are:

- Ear discomfort (ear popping, ear pressure, earache, hearing loss)

- Behavioural or emotional changes (poor sleeping, irritability, underachieving in school, many of the signs and symptoms of ADHD), and speech or language problems.

More often than not, the immediate 'solution' is antibiotics,[45–47] despite the well-published evidence that the routine, repetitive use of antibiotics in treating otitis media increases its recurrence three to sixfold. Eighty per cent or more of this epidemic of ear problems could be avoided simply by identifying and avoiding food allergens, as at least four out of five of these children are food allergic.

What happens is this: the allergic reactions cause the Eustachian tube that drains the middle ear to swell and close. Identify and stop eating allergic foods, and the Eustachian tube will open and drain, and infection and/or fluid build-up will disappear. No more monthly visits to the doctor's office, or prescriptions for antibiotics that don't work very well. It's that simple.

In our opinion, every single child suffering from repeated bouts of otitis media should be tested and treated for food allergy.

▪ Asthma

As we saw in the preceding chapter (see page 43), food allergies often result in diseases of the airways, the most serious of which is asthma.[48] In the UK, 1 in 5 children now have asthma, compared to just 1 in 25 adults – in fact, asthma is now the leading cause of school absenteeism for children under 15.

We've shown how allergic reactions can cause the airways to become irritated or to constrict, leading to a cascade of symptoms that can have sufferers wheezing, coughing, or even fighting to breathe. In children, this can be a real blow to their confidence and leave them in fear of the next attack. But an overreliance on inhalers, as we've seen, isn't the answer. They can be a huge health risk – and if corticosteroids are involved, your child's growth in height can actually be slowed by about an inch a year.

Trying to treat the wheezing and coughing rather than the underlying cause is too limited a solution. We recommend that every child with asthma be checked for food allergy.

■ Sleeping problems and bedwetting

Sleeping problems

Many parents struggle to get their child to sleep, not realizing that food allergies may be making them hyperactive. That glass of milk before bed may make matters worse, not better.

A study of 71 babies, 50 of them poor sleepers, showed that milk is a common allergen in infants. The babies with sleep problems showed raised levels of antibodies to milk, and when milk was eliminated from their diets, their sleep pattern became normal. When milk was then reintroduced to their diets, their sleeplessness returned.[49] In another study, 17 under-fives were referred to a sleep clinic for their continual waking and crying during sleep times. To determine if a food allergy could be contributing to their insomnia, cow's milk was excluded from their diets. Within six weeks, the children were falling asleep more easily, and slept more solidly and for longer – on average, from 5.5 to 13 hours. Reintroducing cow's milk into their diets caused their insomnia to recur.[50]

There can, of course, be other allergies behind sleeplessness, so the best course of action is to have your child tested.

Bed-wetting

Bed-wetting is another problem for families with young children – tens of thousands of them, in fact. Between 10 and 15 per cent of children wet their beds regularly, and 5 per cent of them will still have the problem in adulthood.

Bed-wetting children can be consumed by feelings of guilt and low self-esteem as they see how ever-present piles of laundry and odours of urine affect their parents. Bed-wetters are often reluctant to stay overnight with friends, or engage in a number of activities children normally do. And there can be related problems. ADHD – commonly a food allergic condition – is more prevalent in bed-wetters.[51] So on top of the bed-wetting, many children with the condition have to cope with a range of typical ADHD symptoms (see page 48).

In the early 1990s Dr Joseph Egger – then at London's Great Ormond Street Hospital for Sick Children – studied 21 children with migraines or hyperactivity who were also bed-wetters, and who had previously responded well to a 'few foods' diet (a diet free from the most allergenic foods). He identified which of the foods provoked migraines or hyperactivity in each child and removed these from their diets. The bed-wetting stopped altogether in over half the children and decreased in a further fifth of them.[52]

In our experience, most bed-wetters have hidden food allergies. Allergic reactions can irritate the bladder wall, and as we've seen, also provoke sleep disorders – of which bed-wetting is one. When the food allergy is solved, the child sleeps more restfully, and is able to wake up to make it to the toilet in time.

■ Type 1 diabetes

Diabetes is a chronic disease in which the human body either doesn't produce enough insulin – the hormone that helps regulate blood sugar and turn it into energy – or is unable to use it properly. The high levels of sugar in a diabetic's blood mean they have low energy.

There are two primary types of diabetes. About 90 per cent of diabetics have Type 2, which used to be called 'maturity-onset' diabetes because it usually sets in in adulthood. Type 1 diabetes is always detected in childhood. People with type 1 produce very little or no insulin, and need daily injections of the hormone to prevent their blood sugar levels from getting dangerously high. Hence its other name, 'insulin-dependent' diabetes. In the UK alone, type 1 diabetes affects over 100,000 people and accounts for 8,000 deaths a year.

Type 1 diabetes tends to run in families, suggesting a genetic predisposition to developing it. But its cause is still unknown. So what's the link with food allergy?

In this kind of diabetes, the child's immune system attacks insulin-producing cells in the pancreas. It is therefore classed as an 'auto-immune' disease. There is increasing evidence that what might be happening is that the child becomes allergic to a particular food protein, and that the immune system reacts not only to this, but to a similar protein in the pancreas. This 'cross-reaction' theory is gaining credence and suggests that, in children who may be genetically susceptible to developing the condition, the major trigger might be introducing allergy-provoking foods too early – before the gut and immune system are fully mature.[53-61]

These so-called diabetogenic foods, in order of importance, include:

- Gluten grains

- Soya products[62]

■ Cow's milk.

Growing evidence is linking type 1 diabetes to an allergy to bovine serum albumin (BSA), a substance found in dairy products.[63] Genetically susceptible children who had been breast-fed for at least seven months or exclusively breast-fed for at least three or four months were found to have a significantly decreased incidence of type 1 diabetes, which suggests that another factor is involved. Children who have not been given cow's milk until four months or older also show the same substantially reduced risk. The highest incidence of type 1 diabetes is found in Finland, which is also the world's biggest consumer of dairy products.

Animal studies show that rats bred to be susceptible to diabetes have a much higher risk of getting the disease if their feed contains either milk or wheat gluten. In one study, even the addition of 1 per cent skimmed milk to their diet increased the incidence of type 1 diabetes from 15 to 52 per cent.

Dr Hans-Michael Dosch, Professor of Immunology at Mount Sinai Hospital in New York, identified BSA as the specific factor in dairy produce that increases the risk of diabetes, and showed that it cross-reacted with the cells of the pancreas. He and his fellow researchers theorised that diabetes-susceptible babies introduced to BSA earlier than around four months, a period when the gut wall is immature and more permeable, would develop an allergic response to BSA. As a result, their immune cells would mistakenly destroy not only the BSA molecules but also pancreatic tissue. He went on to show that, of 142 newly diagnosed type 1 diabetic children, 100 per cent had antibodies to BSA, compared to 2 per cent in normal children. Dosch believes that the presence of these anti-BSA antibodies indicates future type 1 diabetes in 80 to 90 per cent of cases.

He also thinks that keeping children off dairy products for at least their first six months halves the risk. BSA can, however, pass from the mother's diet into her milk. So if breastfeeding mothers avoid beef and dairy products, the risk can be completely removed in genetically susceptible children. The current opinion is that about one in four children are genetically susceptible.

International research indicates that early and long-term avoidance of allergenic, 'diabetogenic' foods, combined with a highly varied diet of wholesome and non-allergenic foods, can reduce a diabetic child's need for insulin by as much as two-thirds. So it's well worth having an IgG food allergy test to find out if you or your child are eating any offending foods.

What do I do if my baby is allergic to milk?

Cow's milk allergy is one of the most common in infants and young children, and is notorious for causing a wide variety of allergic symptoms. Identifying cow's milk allergy and removing milk from the diet of an allergic baby may appear easy enough, but deciding what to substitute for it is not. Currently, the two most commonly suggested substitutes are goat's or sheep's milk, and hydrolysed (partially predigested and hypoallergenic) soya or milk protein formulas.

The challenge in all this is that infants allergic to cow's milk may be allergic to other foods and protein formulas, too. Consider this: allergic reactions to other foods, especially to soya, wheat, beef, peanuts and citrus fruits develop in about 50 per cent of proven cow's milk allergic infants.

Moreover, goat's or sheep's milk is not a good substitute for cow's milk in allergic babies. For example, one study of

▶

26 young children with proven milk allergy found all the children were also allergic to goat's milk. Their immune systems couldn't distinguish the cow's milk protein, casein, from goat's or sheep's casein. In spite of this, some doctors continue to recommend goat's milk formulas for babies with cow's milk allergy.

When first commercially introduced, soya formulas were the only available substitute for cow's milk. Today, soya protein formulas are widely used alternatives for babies with proven cow's milk allergy, as well as high-risk allergy-prone infants when human breast milk is not available. However, you need to be aware that up to a third of all cow's milk allergic infants are also allergic to soya protein. You can find this out by giving your child an IgG food allergy test.

Without a doubt, breast milk is best. However, if breast-feeding is not an option, feeding with a hydrolised milk whey formula (milk protein with the highly allergenic milk protein casein removed) is associated with lower incidence of food allergies. There are also other low allergenic milks available in health food stores, such as quinoa milk and almond milk, which are both reasonably high in protein, although they do not contain all the nutrients that specialised milk formulas are enriched with and therefore are not an alternative to breast milk or formula.

5

The Top 20 Common Food Allergens

YOU ARE UNIQUE. That means that what you may or may not be allergic to is individual to you. That being said, after two decades and tens of thousands of IgG allergy tests, it's been found that certain foods are more likely to initiate allergic reactions than others. This does not necessarily mean that the food in question is 'bad' – just that it's bad for you if you react. As you'll see in the next chapter, just about anybody can develop food allergies to the foods they eat most often if their digestive tract (that small football pitch inside you) has become more permeable, allowing undigested food proteins to enter the bloodstream.

Also, as we've seen so far, it is largely the proteins within food that the body's immune system reacts to. For example, some people react to fish but not to fish oil. Others react badly to milk but not to butter. Those with dairy allergies often react worst to low-fat milk, which has a higher relative protein content than full-fat milk, in which the fat actually slows down the absorption of the protein.

The 20 most common food or food group allergens are shown in the box below, in descending order. Of all these foods, by far the most common allergy-provoking substances are dairy products, yeast, eggs and grains, especially wheat.

The Top 20 Common Delayed-onset IgG Food Allergies

1. Cow's milk
2. Wheat gliadin
3. Gluten (gliadin) – found in wheat, rye and barley
4. Yeast
5. Egg whites
6. Cashew nuts
7. Egg yolk
8. Garlic
9. Soya beans
10. Brazil nuts
11. Almonds
12. Corn
13. Hazelnuts
14. Oats
15. Lentils
16. Kiwi fruit
17. Chilli peppers
18. Sesame seeds
19. Sunflower seeds
20. Peanuts

In the sections that follow, we'll explain why it may be unwise for anyone to eat three of the most common allergy-provoking foods – milk, wheat and yeast – on a daily basis. And we'll explain what it is about other common foods that make them more likely than others to provoke allergy in some of us.

■ Milk – a four-letter word?

Whichever way you look at it, cow's milk is consistently the most common food allergen. Classic IgE-based milk allergy is the most common food allergy, and so too is hidden or delayed-onset IgG milk allergy. A myriad of studies have shown that milk-sensitive people have much higher levels of IgG antibodies that target milk proteins than people who are not sensitive to milk.[64-72]

Most cheeses, cream, yoghurt and butter contain milk protein, and it's hidden in all sorts of food. If you check labels, you'll find it's sometimes called simply milk protein, sometimes whey (which is milk protein with the casein removed) and sometimes casein, which is the predominant type of protein – and the most allergenic – in dairy products. You'll be amazed at how many foods contain milk – from bread and cereals to packaged food and crisps. So if you're tested and find you're allergic to milk, you will have to be vigilant with processed foods.

Milk's status as an allergen isn't surprising. This is a highly specific food, containing all sorts of hormones designed for the first few months of a calf's life. It's also a relatively recent addition to the human diet. Approximately 75 per cent of people (25 per cent of people of Caucasian origin and 80 per cent of Asian, Native American or African origin) stop producing lactase, the enzyme that's needed to digest the milk sugar lactose, once they've been weaned – one of many clues that human beings aren't meant to drink cow's milk, at least beyond early childhood.[73] Lactase deficiency or lactose intolerance leads to diarrhoea, bloating, cramping and excess gas.

However, it's not the lactose that causes the allergic reaction. It's the protein. In other words, you can be either lactose intolerant, or milk protein allergic, or both; and in fact, lactose intolerance and milk allergy often occur together.

Of course, most of us have been brainwashed by milk marketers since childhood into believing that milk is practically a wonder food. This can only leave you speculating how half the world, for example most of China and Africa, can survive, let alone thrive, without it. Milk is a reasonably good source of calcium, among other nutrients, but drinking milk certainly isn't the only way, or necessarily the best way, to achieve optimum nutrition. On top of that, it contributes to a wide range of common diseases.

Cow's milk is a major contributing factor to middle-ear infections (otitis media – see also page 53), an allergic disease that affects over a million of our babies and children each year. Milk allergy also contributes to iron deficiency, the most common nutritional deficiency in the world, by impeding the absorption of iron, and damaging the inside lining of the intestines, which causes slow blood leakage and a further loss of iron in red blood cells. In a quarter of people with iron deficiency, anaemia can set in – seen in about 10 per cent of children overall, 30 per cent of children in inner cities, and as many as half of all children in poor countries.

Cow's milk is also one of the top two or three food allergens found in children and adults with poor sleep, asthma, eczema, migraines, rheumatoid arthritis, hyperactivity, bronchitis, more frequent infections and longer hospital stays for premature infants, non-seasonal allergic rhinitis, bed-wetting, so-called growing pains, colic, heartburn, indigestion, chronic diarrhoea, chronic fatigue, hyperactivity, depression, autism, epilepsy (although only in those with concomitant migraines and/or hyperactivity), and perhaps, as we saw above, even type 1 diabetes. If you have ever suffered from any of these conditions, milk should be high on your suspect list for a hidden food allergy. Iain's story bears this out.

case study

Seven-year-old Iain had suffered from chronic insomnia, extreme hyperactivity and asthma all his life. His behaviour was affecting his learning at school. An IgG food allergy test identified that he was allergic to milk. Iain had been in the habit of regularly drinking up to two pints of milk a day.

Within a week of cutting all dairy products from his diet, Iain's mother began to notice a difference in his behaviour. He was less excitable, more settled and could concentrate better. Over the following months, other problems began to reduce significantly. He began sleeping through the night and no longer needed steroid medication for his asthma. On the odd occasion when some milk slips into his diet, some of his behavioural problems and the insomnia return with a vengeance – thankfully, says his mother, only temporarily.

If you are allergic to cow's milk, goat's or sheep's milk are not a viable alternative. They all contain casein, and your immune system is unlikely to be able to distinguish one milk from the other.

Getting enough calcium without milk

If you're allergic to milk, getting the right amount of calcium becomes an issue of particular concern. After all, it is a fact that milk is a good source of both calcium and vitamin D, both of which are needed by the body to build healthy bones. No one who has seen elderly women severely bent over from osteoporosis of the spine can take the issue of calcium loss in the bones lightly. Yet a 1997 study found no connection between teenage consumption of calcium from cow's milk and the risk of bone fractures later on as an adult.[74] Other studies have concluded that the more dairy products a woman consumes, the more likely she will suffer from osteoporotic bone fractures![75–78]

Not all studies have revealed such findings, but the evidence for milk helping to build strong bones is far from clear-cut. The linear idea that bones contain calcium, and milk contains calcium, so milk must be good for the bones, crumbles in the light of recent research published in the *British Medical Journal*. This study shows that supplementing calcium makes no real difference to the risk of osteoporosis.[79] The study gave over 3,000 woman aged 70 and over, all of whom were deemed to be at high risk for osteoporosis, supplements of 1,000mg of calcium and 800ius of vitamin D, or nothing. After two years there was no difference in fracture rate between those supplementing calcium and vitamin D and those who weren't. Despite all this, both the US and UK governments help fund dairy industry campaigns to get kids and teenagers drinking more milk!

The simple truth is that we've become overly obsessed by the role of calcium deficiency in osteoporosis – an attitude that has driven an obsession with drinking that highly allergenic substance, milk. There are plenty of other factors that contribute to poor bone formation, reduced bone density and osteoporosis: high blood pressure; undetected coeliac disease; a diet excessively high in animal protein, including dairy; high caffeine consumption; excessive alcohol; excessive salt and refined sugar; lack of weight-bearing exercise; advancing age; and diets low in nutrients such as vitamins C, D, and K, and/or minerals such as magnesium, manganese, copper, boron and silicon, as well as calcium. Even a lack of onions in your diet may accelerate bone loss!

All these areas are worth looking at in your life. In the meantime, how can you get that calcium? The chart below shows you sources other than dairy products. See how milk products compare to these foods. If you start your day with cereal and soya or rice milk or any other milk fortified with calcium, and a heaped tablespoon of ground seeds, you've already achieved 404mg of calcium. Have a few almonds and a bean dish during the day, with some broccoli, and you're up to 800mg of calcium. That's the equivalent of two and a half glasses of milk. The RDA of calcium for an adult is 800mg, and most decent multivitamins will provide a further 200mg. So, there's no need to go short if you eat a healthy diet free from dairy products, but you do need to know what to eat.

Common sources of calcium: how they compare

Milk – 250 ml = 315 mg calcium
Firm cheese – 50g = 350mg calcium
Yoghurt – 175ml = 275mg calcium

Food	Serving (mg)	Calcium	Rating
Almonds	125mg (½ cup)	(200)	**
Baked beans	250mg (1 cup)	(163)	**
Beet greens, cooked	125mg (½ cup)	(87)	*
Bok choi, cooked	125mg (½ cup)	84	*

▶

Food	Serving (mg)	Calcium	Rating
Brazil nuts	125mg (½ cup)	130	*
Bread, wholewheat or white	1 slice	25	
Broccoli, cooked	125mg (½ cup)	38	
Cauliflower, cooked	125mg (½ cup)	18	
Chickpeas, cooked	250mg (1 cup)	84	*
Dates	60mg (¼ cup)	12	
Figs, dried	4 medium	61	*
Kale, cooked	125mg (½ cup)	103	*
Lentils, cooked	250mg (1 cup)	40	
Nuts, mixed	125mg (½ cup)	48	
Orange	1 medium	52	*
Prunes, dried, uncooked	60mg (¼ cup)	18	
Raisins	60mg (¼ cup)	21	
Red kidney beans, cooked	250mg (1 cup)	(52)	*
Rhubarb, cooked	125mg (½ cup)	(184)	**
Rice, white or brown	125mg (½ cup)	12	
Rice drink (fortified)	250mg (1 cup)	300	***
Salmon, canned with bones	1/2 213g can	225	**
Sardines, canned with bones	1/2 213g can	210	**
Sesame seeds	125mg (½ cup)	(104)	*
Sesame paste (tahini)	30mg (2 tbsp)	(40)	
Shrimps, cooked/canned	70g (12 large)	41	
Soya beans, cooked	125 (½ cup)	(93)	*
Soya drink	250mg (1 cup)	28	
Soya drink (fortified)	250mg (1 cup)	300	***
Spinach, cooked	125mg (½ cup)	(129)	*
Tofu, regular processed*	100g (⅓ cup)	(150)	*
White beans, cooked	250mg (1 cup)	(170)	**

( ) – Calcium from these foods is known to be absorbed less efficiently by the body.

* The calcium content shown for tofu is an approximation based on products available on the market. Calcium content varies greatly from one brand to the other and can be quite low. Tofu processed with magnesium chloride also contains less calcium.

Rating as established according to Canadian Food and Drugs Regulations

* Source of calcium

** Good source of calcium

*** Excellent source of calcium

Source: Health Canada, Canadian Nutrient File, 1993

▪ Wheat, gluten and gliadin – cereal killers?

Your daily bread may be your deadly bread, and you may not even know it. Wheat, some other grains and the cereal proteins gluten and gliadin could be a big factor in any feelings of unwellness you're experiencing.

Hidden risk – coeliac disease

The old view was that about 1 in 5,000 people had coeliac disease, the genetically transferred digestive and malnutrition disorder caused by an extreme allergy to gluten. However, new research shows that gluten allergy affects possibly as many as 1 in 100 normal, symptom-free people, often showing no digestive symptoms at all, and as many as 1 in 10 people with diabetes or thyroid disease.

Go back ten years and coeliac disease was diagnosed by gut biopsy to see if the villi – tiny finger-like protrusions in the intestine walls that aid nutrient absorption – had shrivelled up and flattened. Nowadays, it's most easily diagnosed by a simple blood test called the Ig anti-tissue transglutaminase test, or IgAtTG for short (also available as a home test kit – see Resources). Other tests for coeliacs are discussed on page 93.

When this test was randomly carried out on schoolchildren, it was found to occur in 1 in every 167 so-called normal, healthy children and 1 in every 111 normal, healthy adults.[80] Among those who report gastrointestinal symptoms, it occurs in 1 in 40 children and 1 in 30 adults. Among those who have a father, mother, brother, sister or grandparent with coeliac disease, the risk is 1 in 11. So the condition is far from rare.

However, many more people are allergic to wheat and other gluten grains, but don't have coeliac disease. This is often because their immune systems produce IgG antibodies that attack wheat, or a component of it, producing a whole host of insidious and not immediate symptoms that somehow never develop into full-blown coeliac disease.

So what are the symptoms of gluten allergy? The table on the following page gives the most common ones. Remember, however, that many gluten sensitive people have no digestive symptoms at all. If you have a number of these symptoms, or risk factors, we strongly advise you to get tested (see next chapter).

Common symptoms of gluten allergy

- Upper respiratory tract problems like sinusitis and 'glue ear'
- Fatigue caused by malabsorption of nutrients
- Chronic fatigue syndrome
- Mouth ulcers
- Anaemia
- Osteoporosis
- Weight loss
- Short stature in children
- Iron-deficiency anaemia
- Diarrhoea
- Constipation
- Abdominal bloating
- Crohn's disease
- Diverticulitis
- Depression
- Attention and behavioural problems in children, including ADHD
- Autism.

The trouble with wheat

Wheat is a big staple in our diets. Some 600 million tons of it are eaten every year, and it makes up about half the average person's diet. So the idea that it isn't good for you may be difficult to swallow. However, a look at our history tells a different story.

Species take time to adapt to any new food. Our branch of primates separated from other apes, and became upright, about 4 million years ago. So, we've got a genetic record stretching back 4 million years. Humans started eating gluten grains, at the earliest, 10,000 years ago. So if the history of mankind was condensed into 24 hours, we've been eating gluten grains for, at most, 6 minutes. Some cultures only started eating wheat in the last 100 years – the last 2 seconds. Thanks to advances in DNA research, we now know that humans shrank when they shifted to a grain-eating diet. Our hunter/gatherer ancestors, living on meat, fish and seafood, vegetables, fruit, nuts and seeds, were 5 to 6 inches taller than those early farmers, and had brains 11 per cent bigger.

Recently, it has been discovered that people with gluten allergies have a genetic 'tag' called DQ2 and DQ8, which is common in societies that introduced grains late – notably the northwest of Europe, especially western Ireland, Iceland, Finland and Scandinavia, where grain growing isn't easy. This research is revealing that as many as one in three people in Britain may be allergic to gluten.

Knowing all this, you might wonder why we are eating so much wheat. The answer is simply that bakers the world over love to work with cereals that have a high gluten content (Canadian hard wheat is an international favourite for this reason). The higher the gluten content, the more elastic, malleable, expandable and heat resistant the dough becomes. This results in lighter, softer, more visually attractive, delicious tasting and profitable breads, bagels, pastas, biscuits and pastries.

A worrying trend in the US, where 'low-carb' diets are a craze, is to remove the carbohydrates from wheat products so you're just eating the protein. As this is principally gluten, it's a recipe for disaster for anyone with a hidden gluten allergy. So popular have high-gluten products become in the modern diet that wheat products represent 3 of the top 6 foods, in terms of calories consumed, of both the British and Americans – the other 3 are dairy products. So, what's the alternative?

While gluten is the key protein in wheat, it's also found in rye, barley and oats. In fact, gluten is a name for a family of proteins found in grains. The principal type of gluten in wheat is called gliadin, followed by glutenin,[81] while the main type of gluten in rye is called hirudin, and in barley, secalin, although both also contain some gliadin. These are similar chemically, so a person who is sensitive to wheat is more likely to react to barley than rye. The type of gluten found in oats, however, bears no resemblance to gliadin. Approximately 80 per cent of people diagnosed with coeliac disease don't react to oats.[82–83]

If you suspect you might be gluten-sensitive, you could start by avoiding all gluten grains (wheat, rye, barley and oats) for at least 10 days. Remember, too, that gluten is hidden in many processed foods. If this avoidance diet makes you feel noticeably better, you could then try reintroducing oats, since oats contains no gliadin, and see what happens.

About one in three people tested using an IgG food intolerance test will react to wheat. Of these, 90 per cent will react to gliadin, while 15 per cent will react to barley and 2 per cent to rye. Even fewer react to oats. We think it's well worth getting yourself checked out. It saves a lot of guesswork.

Most people's immune systems, and that may mean you, react to gliadin when it gets into the bloodstream. After all, as we saw above, it's an alien protein that hasn't been around for long in evolutionary terms. Research shows that at least 15 per cent of wheat eaters do have gliadin in their blood. Of course, if you have good genes, don't eat wheat very often, have impeccable digestion and a superhealthy digestive tract, no gliadin is going to get into your bloodstream.

In the box below, you can see which grains contain gluten and which do not. (Note that spelt, kamut and triticale are all forms or hybrids of wheat.)

Gluten Grains	Non-gluten Grains
Wheat	Buckwheat
Spelt	Corn
Rye	Millet
Barley	Maize
Oats (no gliadin)	Rice
Kamut	Quinoa
Triticale	Amaranth

Going gluten-free?

If you have any of the symptoms above, and have proven IgG allergic to wheat gluten and gliadin, it's well worth getting tested for coeliac disease (see page 93). As Pat shows, it's never too late to test.

case study

Pat suffered from unexplained chronic iron-deficiency anaemia, weight loss, fatigue, lower back pain, premature osteoporosis, gastrointestinal bleeding, bloating and loss of appetite. After 35 years of these debilitating symptoms, Pat was diagnosed with coeliac disease – confirmed by both blood tests and biopsy. Within three months of excluding gluten from her diet, her iron levels had normalised and she had achieved a normal body weight.

If, after testing, you prove to be in the 10 per cent of people with gluten or gliadin allergy, or are one of the 1 in 111 apparently healthy adults who actually have coeliac disease, you'll need to give up all the gluten in your diet. If that sounds easy, prepare for a shock.

You will discover that gluten is found in literally thousands of processed, packaged foods. Just go to your local supermarket and start reading labels – there's wheat in soups, sauces, gravies and sausages and hundreds of other unsuspected foods. Soon you will realise just how much our modern food production system relies on gluten, and what a challenge it is to make your diet truly gluten-free.

You will have to begin by avoiding all bread and pasta products, doughnuts, pies and cakes. Biscuits, pancakes, waffles, pizza, bagels, muffins, rolls and baked goods of any kind will have to go, unless clearly and credibly labelled 'gluten free'. Eating in restaurants can also be very challenging. Your best bet is to eat simply – whole foods without sauces, coatings or gravies, such as steamed vegetables, fresh fruits, or simply prepared baked or grilled fish. Be sure to ask your waiter or the chef a lot of questions! It may sound tough, but it's vital: it takes less than half a gram of gluten a day to cause toxic inflammation and cell death in your intestines.

If you'd like to know more about coeliac disease, see Appendix 3; or for an in-depth treatment of this condition and wheat allergy, read *Dangerous Grains* by Dr James Braly and Ron Hoggan.

▪ Yeast – problem on the rise

Yeast, the source of the next most widespread food allergy, is found not only in bread as baker's yeast, but also in soya sauce, beer and, to a lesser extent, wine. Beer and lager are fermented with brewer's yeast. If you've noticed that you feel worse after beer or wine than you do after spirits – the 'cleanest' being vodka – then you may be yeast sensitive.

Does this mean you can't drink? Not at all: it just means you'll need to pick and choose. Stick to spirits, or have a glass of champagne – made by a double-fermentation process, there's much less yeast in it. It's a good idea to limit your consumption of alcohol overall, though. As well as causing allergies in some, alcohol irritates the digestive tract, making it more permeable to undigested food proteins. This increases your chances of developing an allergic reaction to anything, and it's why some people feel at their worst when they eat foods they're allergic to *and* drink alcohol. For example, you might be mildly allergic to wheat and milk and feel fine after either. But when you have both (pasta with cream sauce, for example), plus alcohol, you don't feel great. This combination often will provoke migraine headaches and asthmatic attacks.

Some people think they are allergic to wheat because they feel worse after eating bread. If you've noticed this – perhaps feeling sluggish, tired, bloated or blocked up – but feel fine after pasta, you may not be allergic to wheat, but to the yeast in bread. This is what happened to Janette.

case study

Over seven years, Janette's weight soared by 42lb (19kg) to 189lb (86kg), even though she stuck strictly to a low-calorie diet and took regular exercise. Not only was she heavier than before, but she also felt constantly tired and uncomfortably bloated after meals, particularly when she'd eaten bread. An IgG food allergy test showed she was allergic to yeast, milk, corn, soya, and haricot and kidney beans. Simply by avoiding these foods, Janette lost 28lb in five months!

Getting tested, in short, is the only way to be sure.

■ Nuts and beans – seeds of destruction?

Nuts and beans are part of the same food family, along with fruit pips. Essentially, they're all seeds. The most common individual allergens in this group are, in descending order: cashew nuts, soya beans, Brazil nuts, almonds, hazelnuts and peanuts. You can react to one and not others, but if you do react to a member of this family there's a greater chance that you'll react to another. Coffee and chocolate, both of which originate as beans, are also members of this family.

The most common immediate-onset, IgE allergy-causing foods are peanuts and tree nuts (such as almonds, walnuts, pecans and cashews), according to the US-based Food Allergy and Anaphylaxis Network (FAAN). About 1.5 million people in the US and a possible 300,000 in the UK are allergic to peanuts (not a true nut, but a legume – in the same family as beans, peas and lentils). Half of those allergic to peanuts are also allergic to tree nuts, and often sunflower and sesame seeds. Research is also reporting that soya allergy is rapidly increasing, approaching the incidence of peanut allergy in Europe and the US.

Unlike allergies to other foods like milk and eggs, children generally don't outgrow allergies to peanuts or nuts. But over time, they should become experienced at avoiding the foods that make them ill.

Recognising and diagnosing a nut allergy

The first signs of an immediate allergic reaction can be a runny nose, a skin rash all over the body or a tingly tongue. The symptoms may quickly become more severe and include signs of anaphylaxis (a sudden, potentially severe allergic reaction involving various systems in the body), such as difficulty breathing, swelling of the throat or other parts of the body, a rapid drop in blood pressure, and dizziness or unconsciousness. Other possible symptoms include hives, tightness of the throat, a hoarse voice, nausea, vomiting, abdominal pain, diarrhoea and lightheadedness.

To a person with no allergies, seeing someone else experiencing anaphylaxis can be just as scary as it is for the allergic person. What's more, anaphylaxis can happen just seconds after exposure to the allergen. It can involve various areas of the body (the skin, respiratory tract, gastrointestinal tract and cardiovascular system), and can be mild to fatal. The annual incidence of anaphylactic reactions is small – about 30 per 100,000 people – although people with asthma, eczema or hay fever are at greater risk of having them.

Obviously, babies can't tell their parents when their tummies hurt or their throats itch, so diagnosing food allergies early in a child's life can be difficult. We therefore generally recommend that parents refrain from giving their children peanut butter or other peanut or nut products until after they're two years old. If there's a family history of food allergies, parents should wait until the child is three. And many doctors recommend that their pregnant patients – especially those with food allergies – keep the lid on the peanut butter jar until after the baby is born and they've finished breastfeeding.

If your doctor suspects your child might have a peanut or nut allergy, he or she will probably refer you to an allergy specialist for further testing because, as we've seen, the reactions can be very dangerous, even fatal. The allergy specialist will ask you and your child questions, such as how often your child has the reaction, how quickly symptoms start after eating a particular food, and whether any family members have allergies or conditions like eczema and asthma.

■ Soya – friend or foe?

Soya is something of a byword for health these days. Soya protein, isoflavones (plant-based compounds found in soya products) and fibre have been found to reduce the risk of developing menopausal problems, breast and prostate cancer, and cardiovascular risk – probably by reducing 'bad' LDL cholesterol, triglycerides (blood fats) and other culprits. As such, it could benefit many type 1 diabetics who are concerned about the high risk of coronary artery disease their condition carries.

This array of benefits has prompted most nutrition experts to jump on the soya bandwagon. And there's more. Along with all soya's remarkable disease-fighting attributes, vegetarians claim that it's a healthy and 'ethical' milk and meat substitute. So where's the problem?

As with any food, if you're allergic to it, it's bad news. And soya allergies and soya-induced illnesses are unfortunately very common. With soya consumption rapidly on the rise (tripling over the last three years as it appears in more and more processed foods, from hamburgers, sausages and salad dressings to chicken nuggets and breakfast cereals), there is an escalating increase in reports of allergic reactions. The reason for the explosion in soya allergy isn't completely known, but one proposed explanation is that GM soya is more likely to cause allergies, and GM soya use has risen sharply in recent years.

The adverse effects can be very serious. If babies allergic to soya are introduced to it early in life (perhaps as an alternative to formula milk if they weren't breast-fed), that can actually increase the risk of developing type 1 diabetes. Along with wheat, milk casein and perhaps BSA (the other protein in milk linked to diabetes), soya is considered a major diabetes-causing food.

Like peanuts, soya can also induce anaphylaxis in people severely allergic to it. In fact, soya and peanuts often cross-react – an allergy to peanuts is associated with a disproportionate degree of soya allergy, and vice versa.

By the way, soya and other beans and lentils are high in a type of carbohydrate called glucosides. These are quite hard for most of us to digest, but not for the bacteria within our guts. The net result is that they produce gas and possible bloating. But this does not necessarily mean that you are allergic. First, try chewing them more thoroughly. There's nothing like inadequate chewing of beans and lentils for producing gas. You could also go to a health food store and buy a digestive enzyme containing amyloglucosidase (also called glucoamylase), which helps you digest beans. If this relieves the embarrassing symptoms, there's no reason to assume you are allergic, unless other allergic symptoms – which for soya can include sinusitis and rhinitis – remain.

If you aren't allergic, it's good to know that some soya products are easier to handle than others (the Far East is awash in soya, after all). Soya beans themselves contain a number of 'anti-nutrients' that makes them hard to digest and also impede the absorption of other nutrients. Enzyme inhibitors in the beans, for instance, get in the way of the body's digestion of protein and phytic acid, which results in reduced absorption and bioavailability of iron and zinc. Soya is also high in lectins, which can irritate the gut; it's likely, in fact, that soya allergy is really a soya lectin allergy. But some soya products are low in lectins: fermented soya foods such as miso, natto or tempeh have a fraction of the amount. So too does tofu. Some brands of soya milk also have low levels of these substances.

If you are considering a soya-based diet, perhaps because you're a vegan or are allergic to milk, our advice is first to get tested with an IgG food allergy test.

Eggs – a scrambled tale

Like soya, eggs are a good source of protein, and also contain other important nutrients such as phospholipids, which are vital for the brain. Also like soya, eggs can provoke allergic reactions. These are particularly common in children. In one study of 107 children with dermatitis, 92 were found to be allergic to egg white.[84] Egg allergy is certainly worth suspecting if you have either eczema or dermatitis, and eliminating eggs from the diet of children prone to eczema has proven effective.[85]

In another study investigating 156 children with the symptom of swollen lips, half were found to be allergic to egg white.[86] Egg white allergy is common, causing both immediate-onset IgE-mediated reactions (wheezing, skin rashes and so on) as well as delayed IgG reactions. Reactions to egg white are much more common than to egg yolk, almost certainly because of a type of protein in egg white called ovomucoid. If this is removed from egg white, most people stop reacting.[87] Eggs also contain certain enzyme inhibitors.[88]

It is possible that egg allergy is more common because it, like milk, is very often introduced early into children's diets. Egg allergy is less common in adults.

■ Garlic, chilli and kiwi fruit – pungent peril

The health benefits of garlic have been known for centuries, but remember – we are each unique, and this pungent bulb doesn't suit everybody. If you do test allergic to garlic, also be suspicious of onions, since they come from the same food family. Another common culinary allergen is chilli and, as it's part of the same family as cayenne and paprika, be wary of these if you find you're allergic. Of all the fruits, the most commonly allergenic has been found to be the kiwi fruit. (But obviously, don't give up these delectable vitamin-rich fruits unless you've tested positive for them in an allergy test!)

While this trio are among the most common to come up positive on an allergy test, it's important to recall that food allergies are unique to individuals. For example, in one trial testing 150 people with IBS, 23 people were found to be allergic to the same foods as another patient, but the remainder, that's 127 people, or 85 per cent, had unique test results. In this trial, only one person failed to react to *any* of the top five allergenic foods.[89]

If this trial is anything to go by, it means that the chances you may be reacting to 1 of the top 5 foods are high – but also that the chances you react to *only* 1 of the top 5 are very small indeed. That's why we recommend you get yourself properly tested.

6

Diagnosing Your Food Allergy

As WE EXPLAINED in Chapter 2, there are two main kinds of food allergy: the immediate-onset, Type 1, IgE antibody-based allergy, and the delayed-onset, Type 3, IgG antibody-based allergy. Here's the lowdown on how to test for both.

▪ IgE testing

Doctors use different kinds of tests to identify this much rarer form of food allergy. When using skin testing, the doctor or nurse applies a dilute solution containing a food extract to the skin – often on the back or forearm. The skin is then scratched or punctured, allowing the food to penetrate the surface. If the person has an IgE allergy to that food, a positive reaction will take the form of a red bump resembling a mosquito bite, which appears in 15 to 20 minutes.

There is also a blood test, popularly known as the IgE RAST (radioallergosorbent) test, which is of about the same diagnostic value as the skin test, and its spin-off, the IgE MAST test. They both measure serum levels of food-specific IgE antibodies. Skin tests and IgE RAST or MAST tests *only* detect IgE food allergies, not the IgG type.

In our opinion, the best test for IgE allergies is the IgE ELISA test. ELISA (enzyme linked immunosorbent assay) is a laboratory technique also used for IgG food allergy testing. Exactly how it works is explained on page 87. The ELISA test is available from any allergy specialist, if you've been referred by your doctor, or from a number of laboratories listed in Resources on page 170. However, don't forget that IgE food allergies are far rarer than IgG food allergies, making this a less useful test unless you have severe and immediate reactions to food.

■ IgG testing

If you are chronically ill but have no firm diagnosis of the cause, a vital first step on the road to optimum health is to suspect that a delayed-onset IgG food allergy may be involved. The crucial second step is to accurately identify and eliminate the relevant food allergens.

It should come as no surprise, however, that diagnosing delayed-onset food allergies has been fraught with seemingly insurmountable challenges. The symptoms of this kind of allergy show up gradually, in many forms and in many regions of the body, and can be triggered by a number of commonly eaten foods. The picture is muddied further because eating the allergen can actually make you feel better temporarily – a phenomenon sometimes known as food addiction – and may not even provoke an allergic reaction every time you eat it. The sufferers' tales of woe about visits to one doctor after another are commonplace. Here are a couple of classic quotes we've often heard:

case studies

I was skin tested for food allergy and nothing showed up allergic, only to be told later that skins tests were inaccurate tests for most food allergies.

Once I was tested and found I was allergic to oranges, but not to wheat. The next month I took another test which said I was allergic to wheat but not to oranges. That's when I gave up.

How IgG testing evolved

For decades, the focus in this field was on 'true' food allergies – namely, the IgE immediate-onset kind – and the diagnostic tool of choice was the skin test (see page 84). But skin testing and IgE RAST blood testing don't work when it comes to detecting IgG food allergies.

It wasn't until the 1980s that published research began to demonstrate that a fundamental mechanism behind IgG food allergy was the penetration of large molecules of incompletely digested food through a leaky intestinal lining into the bloodstream. As food allergens enter the bloodstream, we were being told, IgG antibodies, not IgE, were forming against them.

As we saw in Chapter 2, IgG antibodies bind to the allergens, forming food allergen-antibody immune complexes. These immune complexes circulate throughout the body, and if not gobbled up by the detoxifying immune cells called macrophages, they will penetrate the walls of small blood vessels in various vulnerable sites in the body. Once firmly entrenched, immune complexes become sources of constant irritation, inflammation, and, ultimately, dysfunction and destruction of body tissues. Diseases such as food allergy-induced rheumatoid arthritis can then develop.

Since the gut lining never functions perfectly as a barrier at the best of times, the big difference between a food allergy sufferer and a non-allergic person appears to be the amount of partially digested food that reaches their bloodstream, and how well their immune system clears these allergens from circulation. If a lot of these foods get in over time, and kickstart the formation of many immune complexes, the person will inevitably begin to suffer from an IgG food allergy.

In the IgG test, a sample of blood is drawn and tested for the presence of IgG antibodies formed against foods in your diet. You can now obtain home test kits like the one shown on the following page from nutritionists, health clinics, some chemists and some doctors, as well as by mail order. They contain a simple, almost painless device to obtain the pinprick of blood.

If you choose to do your own IgG ELISA test at home, you might want to get someone else to get the blood sample; although it doesn't hurt, it can be easier if you avert your eyes! Ask them to prick your finger on the side, which has fewer nerve endings than the pad. You then place a tiny column of absorbent material against the drop of blood. You send this off to the laboratory by first class or registered post, and provided it gets there within 72 hours (three days), it's completely accurate.

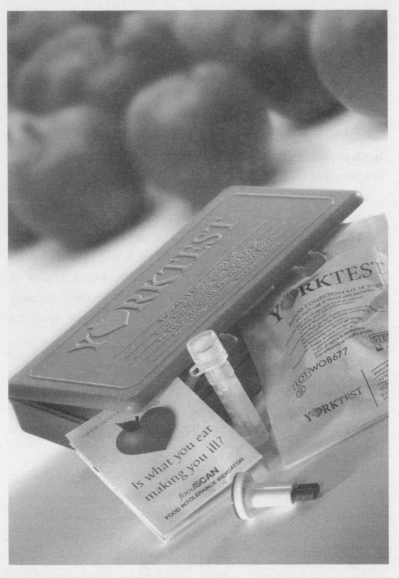

Home test kit, blood collection

Depending on the lab, they can test the blood sample simultaneously against 100 or more foods. The blood is then exposed to tiny containers or wells, each containing a different food protein (see below).

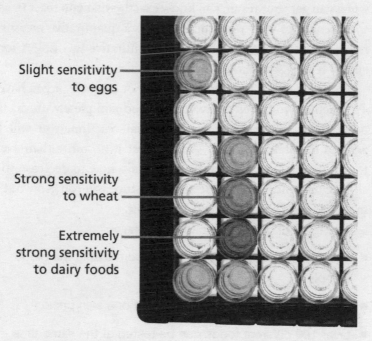

Slight sensitivity to eggs

Strong sensitivity to wheat

Extremely strong sensitivity to dairy foods

Petri dish panel marked up

In the panel above you can see which food proteins have caused a reaction, some more than others. If your blood serum contains abnormally high levels of IgG antibody against a particular food, it means you are allergic to that food. When this happens, as we've seen, the antibody and protein form a complex. The more complexes, the greater the density of the solution becomes. A light is then shone through the containers and the tests results are read and recorded by computerised laboratory equipment.

The ELISA test measures degrees of reaction, which are graded from +1 to +4, with +4 being the strongest reaction. So when you get your result, you know exactly what you react to and the strength of your reaction. As this is a quantitative measurement, this kind of testing is called quantitative IgG ELISA food allergy testing. You should accept no other.

A sample report is shown opposite. For example, if you have a +3 reaction, you need to avoid the food completely. If, on the other hand, you have only a marginal reaction, you will be advised to rotate that food – that is, eat it no more than every fourth day. In the next chapter we explain how to decrease your allergic tendency and reverse allergies, since you can grow out of most IgG food allergies if you know how.

The IgG ELISA test has many advantages:

- You don't have to fast overnight before taking the blood sample

- It is relatively painless, involving just one skin prick

- Over 100 different foods can be tested at the same time

- It is largely an automated test, so if performed with the appropriate lab quality controls, it is accurate and reproducible

- It can be done with blood samples sent through the post, as long as the sample reaches the lab within 72 hours after taking the blood sample.

The IgG ELISA test represents a step forward in the field of food allergy testing. It addresses the enormously prevalent problem of foodSCAN 113 in-depth test : 05/12345 EXAMPLE2

Y♥RKTEST

Client Name : Mr Example Results

Test Date : Friday, 26 August 2005

	AVOID	ROTATE	NO REACTION
Grains	Wheat +2		Barley Buckwheat Corn (Maize) Gluten (Gliadin) Millet Oat Rice Rye
Dairy	Cows Milk +3 Egg White +1		Egg Yolk
Meats			Beef Chicken Duck Lamb Pork Turkey
Fish			Crustacean Mix Mollusc Mix Oily Fish Mix Plaice / Sole Salmon / Trout Tuna White Fish Mix
Vegetables			Asparagus Aubergine Avocado Carrot Celery Cucumber Haricot Bean Kidney Bean Lentils Lettuce Mushroom Mustard Mix Onion Pea Peppers (Capsicum) / Paprika Potato Soya Bean Spinach String Bean
Nuts		Almond Brazil Cashew	Coconut Hazelnut Peanut Walnut

Printout of an example of an allergy test result

delayed food allergy head-on, and removes the barriers of inaccuracy and poor reproducibility that continue to plague many competing tests. It is our test of choice for diagnosing delayed-onset food allergies.

Consider the case of Patrick Webster, otherwise known as Mr Sneezy because he holds the world record for sneezing in the *Guinness Book of World Records*. The IgG ELISA test turned his life around completely.

case study

Patrick Webster's sneezing (non-seasonal allergic rhinitis) began when he was 17, and for the next 35 years of his life averaged roughly 1 sneeze every 2 minutes – that's 600 to 700 sneezes per day or 220,000 sneezes a year, amounting to about 7 million sneezes. So in the end, he had sneezed without interruption for 12,775 days! His relentless sneezing led to fatigue from lack of sleep, and forced him to retire early. Steroid therapy prescribed by his doctors has given him osteoporosis.

Webster finally heard about IgG food allergy testing. His test results revealed that he was allergic to oats, almonds, hazelnuts, milk, cheese, egg yolk and tomatoes. He was not only a big cheese and milk consumer, but in addition, every morning of his adult life, he prepared his own muesli consisting of oats, almonds, Brazil nuts and cow's milk. When he eliminated the muesli and other offending foods, his sneezing stopped and has not returned. For the first time in 35 years, Patrick is totally free of sneezing and nasal congestion and sleeps restfully through the night.

▪ Screening for and diagnosing coeliac disease

We first looked at coeliac disease – a digestive disorder caused by extreme allergy to gluten – in Chapters 3 and 5. Approximately 6 million people in Britain are allergic to gluten cereals – wheat and its hybrids and variants triticale, spelt and kamut; and rye, barley and oats. One in 30 will go on to develop coeliac disease. If you do prove IgG (or IgE) sensitive to grains and gluten or gliadin, we recommend you also get tested for coeliac disease. (For more details on this disease, which we recommend you read if you are allergic to wheat, see Appendix 3.)

Many doctors regard the small-bowel biopsy as the 'gold standard' for the diagnosis of coeliac disease. It is commonly an outpatient procedure performed by a specialist. A long tube is inserted through the mouth, oesophagus, stomach and finally into the small intestine, where several biopsies of mucosa lining are taken. A pathologist looking for the characteristic lesions of coeliac disease studies this tissue under a microscope.

As you can see, this procedure is an expensive and inconvenient diagnostic tool. Many doctors and their patients are understandably reluctant to have it performed unless there is very good reason for doing so.

This is where modern laboratory science comes into play. Several antibody blood tests are currently being used with great success to help distinguish people who are likely candidates for coeliac disease from those who aren't. As a result, many fewer unnecessary biopsies are being performed – saving in both costs and patients' suffering.

Since gliadin appears to be the key offending protein to which coeliacs react, testing to see whether a person is producing antibodies to gliadin can be used to screen for coeliac disease. While we've been talking a lot about IgG antibodies, there's another kind of antibody, called IgA; and often people with coeliac disease produce anti-gliadin IgA antibodies as well as anti-gliadin IgG antibodies. When you have an IgG food allergy test, one of the 100 or so foods you'll be tested for will be gliadin, so you'll have this information already.

Both the IgG and IgA tests are used to screen for coeliac disease. The tests are done together in order to maximise the sensitivity of the screening – that is, to ensure that if you have coeliac disease, one or both of the tests will pick it up well over 90 per cent of the time. However, there is a problem with these tests. Even if you don't have coeliac disease, one of the tests may still come up positive. You may be gliadin allergic, but not have coeliac disease. Clearly, another, more specific screening test needs to be done.

The answer to the dilemma, at least at the moment, is the IgA anti-endomysium test. It is a more expensive and sophisticated screening test for coeliac disease. Due to its expense, it is usually performed after one or both of the less expensive anti-gliadin antibody tests come back positive. It's more accurate, and if you have coeliac disease, it comes up positive for IgA antibodies nearly 100 per cent of the time. If you don't have coeliac disease, it will come back negative approximately 95 per cent of time.

A new test may soon replace this one: the IgA anti-tissue transglutaminase test, or IgAtTG, also known as the TGA ELISA. This measures anti-transglutaminase IgA antibodies in human serum. Like the anti-endomysium assay, it is brought into play when either or both of the anti-gliadin antibody tests are positive. Studies published in Europe and the US confirm that the TGA is equivalent in accuracy to the anti-endomysium test.[90] If positive, it is very likely that you have coeliac disease, and without question a follow-up intestinal biopsy is indicated for final confirmation. Our prediction is that the TGA will soon replace the anti-endomysium assay and may even replace small bowel biopsies. Ask your doctor to run the TGA or anti-endomysium tests if you suspect you have coeliac disease.

7

Why Allergies Develop and How to Prevent or Reverse Them

BY NOW, WE HOPE you will have decided to have a proper food allergy test to find out whether you have IgG or possibly IgE food allergies. But you might be feeling mixed emotions about it: excitement, because you could be pinpointing the source of your ill health – and anxiety, because you feel a sense of loss about giving up favourite foods.

The good news is that you can grow out of most food allergies. While coeliac disease and IgE-based food allergies are fixed and permanent for life, most food allergies only involve IgG antibodies, and your immune system can 'unlearn' its IgG sensitivities. If you avoid a food you are currently IgG sensitive to for three to four months, there will be no more IgG antibodies left tagged for that food and the immune cells producing food-specific IgG antibodies appear to lose interest in doing so over time. This means you won't react allergically to that food when it's reintroduced.

Why not? It's because immune cells that produce IgG antibodies don't pass their 'memory' on to the next generation. They forget. Also, there are things you can do right now to decrease your sensitivity to food allergens. The way to reverse your food allergies is best understood by seeing how you developed them in the first place.

▪ High-risk eating

Have you ever wondered whether the food you eat actually wants to be eaten? In many cases it appears that it doesn't. Most food plants try their best to protect themselves from predators – with spikes, thorns and chemical toxins. The idea that everything in a food is 'good' is far from the truth. Most foods contain numerous natural toxins as well as beneficial nutrients.

Even foods that are obviously designed to be eaten can have this characteristic. For example, many fruits rely on animals eating them, so their seed can be spread in a ready-made manure bed – and thus widen their territory. However, the fruit has to protect itself from unwanted scavengers such as bacteria, viruses or fungi that will simply rot the seed. So some seeds are hard to crack and toxic, such as apricot kernels, which contain cyanide compounds. For protective reasons, wild food contains a massive and often selective chemical arsenal to ward off specific foes. Food and us have been fighting for survival since the beginning of time.

Our survival technique does have a few holes in it, though. Omnivores like us have a high-risk/high-return strategy, as far as food is concerned. We try different foods and if we don't immediately get sick, then it's okay to eat it. But this shortsighted test has failed us, many times. Indeed, even today, the average Western diet kills many people in the long run – although most of us are foraging in supermarkets rather than fields and woods.

■ Why food allergies are on the rise

Before we show you how best to reduce your allergic potential, it's important to understand why food allergies are on the increase. Over the past 20,000 years, people have changed very little – and genetically, not at all. The same, however, cannot be said of our diets.

Many of today's killer diseases, from diabetes to heart disease, have arisen because our unchanging genetic constitution has collided head-on with a radical change in diet. Take a close look at this comparison between what our ancestors were eating 20,000 years ago and today's diet:

Stone-Age Diet	Today's Diet
0% of carbohydrates as cereal grains	75% of carbohydrate as grains
Favourite drinks: mother's milk, water	Fizzy drinks, coffee, tea, alcohol and cow's milk
Great variety of fruits and vegetables eaten	8 to10 foods make up 80% of daily calories (dairy, wheat, refined sugars, fried potatoes)

Today we are drinking more high-sugar, fizzy drinks than water! Times have clearly changed. Are we becoming more food allergic simply because we are eating the wrong foods? When you consider that cow's milk, grains and yeast are all essentially 'new' foods in our human diet, this simplistic idea makes sense. Eating a monotonous diet of high-risk allergy foods is certainly part of the reason why food allergies are on the increase.

Consider the top nine foods eaten in the US, rated by the number of calories consumed annually, as reported by the US Department of Agriculture:

1 Full-fat cow's milk

2 2 per cent-fat cow's milk

3 Processed American cheese

4 White (wheat) bread

5 White (wheat) flour

6 Rolls (wheat)

7 Refined sugar, which accounts for 15 to 21 per cent of all calories

8 Cola

9 Beef mince.

Notice the absence of fruits and vegetables in this list. Notice also that dairy and wheat (gluten) products make up the top six foods. Recall that allergies to cow's milk and wheat are two of the most commonly reported. By eating these foods day in and day out, it's clear why so many people suffer from chronic food allergies over an entire lifetime. But it doesn't completely explain the phenomenon of food allergy.

Let's take a look at some other known factors than increase your chances of developing allergy and, if solved, will reduce your allergic potential:

- Increased intestinal permeability (leaky gut)

- Poor digestion

- Dysbiosis (lack of healthy gut bacteria)

- Lack of nutrients from poor diet

- Not being breast-fed

- Excessively clean environments during infancy and early childhood

- Use of antacids or antibiotics

- Having a parent with allergies

- Non-steroidal anti-inflammatory drugs (NSAIDs)

- Drinking alcohol

- Cross-reactions.

■ The top food allergy promoters

Now let's examine each of these factors in detail. We'll also look more closely at addiction to problem foods.

Have you got leaky gut syndrome?

An obvious place to start in unravelling the true cause of allergies is the digestive tract. After all, the lining of the gut is the first point of contact between foods and the immune system. Did you know that the intestinal lining alone is estimated to contain more immune cells and produce more antibodies than any other organ in the body? Hardly surprising, then, that the intestinal lining and its immune system is an absolutely crucial defence against food allergens and infections.

Normally, the inner lining of your small intestine serves as a highly selective barrier against your internal environment, preventing the entry of potentially harmful toxins, microbes and incompletely digested foods from the gut into blood circulation in much the same way that a bouncer keeps the riff-raff out of an exclusive club – which just happens to be your body. At the same time, this lining selectively allows the passage of important vitamins, minerals, amino acids, essential fatty acids and other nutrients. It permits properly digested food protein, carbohydrates and fats to easily gain entry into the bloodstream.

The trouble starts when this lining becomes more permeable or 'leaky'. Food particles can then enter the blood, and the immune system is exposed to proteins not on the guest list, so to speak, triggering an allergic reaction. Recent research shows that people with food allergies do tend to have leaky gut walls.[91] This might explain why frequently eaten foods are more likely to cause a reaction.

There are many reasons why our modern-day diet might lead to leaky gut. Consumption of alcohol, the frequent use of painkiller drugs such as aspirin, antibiotic use, a deficiency in essential fatty acids or a gastrointestinal infection or infestation (such as candidiasis) are all possible contributors to leaky gut syndrome. If any of these apply to you, they'll need to be corrected in order to reduce your sensitivity to foods.

More, eating foods you're allergic to is another major contributor to a leaky gut. That's right: hidden food allergies encourage more food allergies. So if you're wheat allergic and don't know it – and most people don't – it's probably making your digestive tract more permeable by irritating this inner skin every time you eat wheat. As a consequence, you may develop other food allergies too.

A lack of key nutrients such as glutamine, vitamin A, essential fats or zinc can also prevent proper integrity of the gut wall. More on these later because increasing your intake of key nutrients such as these can decrease your allergic potential.

You are what you digest

Food allergens also tend to pass through the digestive tract incompletely digested. This is because the digestive tract's natural tendency is to try to fend off any substance it perceives as harmful or toxic. So it attaches antibodies to the allergen to try, often successfully, to eliminate the food before it can pass into the bloodstream. The food passes out in the stool partially digested at best – and with it go the nutrients. This is one reason why some people with IBS can get diarrhoea from eating foods they are allergic to.

The end result is sub-optimal nutrition. So it can be said that the first basic requirement of optimum nutrition is a diet free of food allergens.

Developing food allergies becomes even more likely in people who don't produce enough of the right digestive enzymes. You release a staggering 10 litres of digestive juices, hopefully rich with digestive enzymes, into your stomach and intestines every day! Much of this fluid is reabsorbed. But if you lack sufficient enzymes, large amounts of big, undigested food molecules are reaching the gut wall. One research study of people with a sensitivity to man-made chemicals showed that 90 per cent of them produced inadequate amounts of digestive enzymes, compared with 20 per cent of healthy controls.

Later on we'll tell you how supplementing digestive enzymes can have amazing effects on reducing your allergic potential. Zinc supplementation can also be helpful, as a deficiency in this mineral is extremely common among allergy sufferers. Zinc is not only needed for protein digestion, but is also essential for the production of hydrochloric (stomach) acid in the stomach – and without enough stomach acid, you can't digest anything.

Beneficial bacteria – the inside story

Inside the intestines there is a carefully balanced world of 'friendly' and potentially 'unfriendly' bacteria. The 180 friendly, health-promoting strains of bacteria are called probiotics. They include at least nine strains of *Bifidobacteria* and 64 of *Lactobacillus* bacteria.

Probiotic bacteria have many scientifically proven benefits, including:

- Preventing and treating food allergy

- Alleviating intestinal inflammation

- Preventing abnormal gut leakiness or permeability

- Preventing and reversing diarrhoea caused by antibiotics, food allergy and infections

- Suppressing IgE antibody production

- Protecting against or reducing the number of food allergy-provoking candida yeast infections (candidiasis).[92]

Much depends on that balance of probiotics with 'bad' bacteria in the gut, however. If you were introduced to the wrong foods too early in life, or had a poor diet as a child or adult, perhaps with too high a sugar intake or alcohol consumption, or have overused antibiotics and other prescription drugs, it's easy to become deficient in probiotic bacteria, leaving room for disease-causing microbes to take over and dominate. As a result, your digestive tract may become prone to inflammation, leaving your gut leakier and impairing digestion.

Probiotic supplements can help to reverse this imbalance.[93] For example, a Finnish study found breast-fed infants with eczema and cow's milk allergy improved significantly when their mothers were given probiotic bacteria supplements. The report concluded by stating, 'By alleviating intestinal inflammation, [probiotic supplements] may act as a useful tool in the treatment of food allergy.'[94] We'll explain later how to use probiotic supplements to restore your healthy gut bacteria and reduce your allergic potential.

Why breast really is best

Not so long ago, every mother breast-fed her baby – as otherwise, they would die. Human breast milk is a treasurehouse of essential nutrients and immune factors that help infants thrive naturally until they're ready to eat whole foods on their own. But as breastfeeding has declined during the past century, the prevalence of childhood allergies has increased dramatically.

The scientific literature stretching back over the last 30 years is clear. It strongly suggests that exclusive breastfeeding during the first four to six months of life delays by years the appearance and likelihood of food allergies, including:

- Otitis media (middle ear infection and fluid in the middle ear)

- Coeliac disease (gluten sensitivity)

- Wheezing illnesses, like asthma and chronic bronchitis

- Chronic diarrhoeal diseases

- Autoimmune diseases.

So the bottom line is: if at all possible, exclusively breastfeed your baby for at least six months in order to prevent or delay the appearance of food allergies and associated diseases. The sad truth is that very few mothers are heeding this advice. In the UK, 2 out of 3 mothers introduce their children to solids before the age of 4 months. In the US, 2 out of 3 mothers quit breastfeeding their babies entirely at 6 months.

They may not realise that breastfeeding protects their own health as well as their babies'. Research from China, published in the *American Journal of Epidemiology*, shows that women who breastfeed their babies for two years have 50 per cent less incidence of breast cancer compared to women who breast-fed for only 1–6 months.[95] Breastfeeding also greatly reduces the chances of the mother developing mastitis, and of their babies developing chronic diarrhoea (which can be dangerous or even fatal in young children) and respiratory infections.[96]

While breastfeeding is brilliant health insurance, the mother's diet obviously affects breast milk – and with it, the chances of their baby developing allergies. Breast-fed children of mothers who eat a diet high in saturated fats, for instance, have a 16 per cent higher risk of developing allergies, says Dr Ulla Hoppu from Finland, who studied 114 breast-fed babies.[97] Nearly a quarter of this group of infants became sensitised to common allergens by the age of one, most commonly to eggs, milk, wheat and cats.

So how does breast milk do the job of protecting babies from allergy? It has been found that complex proteins and amino acids in breast milk are key to the task. If levels of the organic compounds spermine and spermidine are low in breast milk, the child fed on it will have an 80 per cent chance of developing an allergy. Adding these compounds to formula feed also reduces risk of developing allergy.[98] Breast milk is also higher in brain-friendly phospholipids and omega-3 fats, as long as the mother is eating oily fish and eggs, and ideally supplementing omega-3 fish oils. These fats are not only vital for the brain; they are also essential building materials for healthy gut membranes, which means fewer allergy-provoking food proteins can get through.

Are we too clean?

Paradoxically, an overemphasis on hygiene and a germ-free environment during infancy and early childhood may also contribute to food allergies later in life. According to several recent studies, there is growing scientific evidence that too much emphasis on cleanliness and sterile childhood environments may be associated with as high as a 225 per cent increased risk of developing allergies.

So it seems that exposure to germs early on may bring a degree of protection from childhood and adult food allergies. Surveys have found that children with the highest incidence of infections during infancy or early childhood – that is, living in the least hygienic surroundings – have the lowest incidence of food and airborne allergies later on. If subsequent studies bear this out, we may have to re-evaluate our obsession with the mop and bucket, and conclude that our kids may be, heaven forbid, too clean!

Antacids and antibiotics – bad medicine?

A new study by Austrian researchers indicates that the frequent use of antacids may produce food allergies. The study, headed by Professor Erika Jensen-Jarolim at the University of Vienna, involved approximately 300 people and found that those given antacid pills started to develop food allergy symptoms, while those taking placebos did not. The scientists said that antacid medications may interfere with digestion, thereby causing food to enter one's intestines before it is fully broken down, and so triggering an attack.[99]

A similar effect was found in children given antibiotics early in life. Researchers from the Henry Ford Hospital in Detroit, Michigan, found that children who receive antibiotics within their first six months significantly increase their risk of developing allergies.[100] The researchers found that compared to children not given antibiotics in that time, these children were almost twice as likely to develop asthma, allergies to pets, ragweed, grass and dust mites by the age of seven. The study also showed the youngsters were less susceptible to these effects if they lived with at least two dogs or cats in their first year.

The gene factor

You can inherit allergies – at least the immediate-onset IgE kind.[101] If both your parents have this kind of allergy, there is a 75 per cent chance that you will, too. If only one parent has, your odds are a 30 to 40 per cent chance.[102] Pregnant women who suffer from allergies have been found to be more likely to have babies who develop allergies and asthma, according to a five-year study funded by the British Lung Foundation and Asthma UK. The researchers, however, found that it is possible to minimise that risk by reducing a woman's exposure to allergens while she is pregnant. Dr Jill Warner, who headed the research at Southampton General Hospital, said: 'Our research shows that mothers can influence whether their baby develops sensitisation to allergies. Controlling the mothers' reactions to allergens, especially during the second and third trimesters of pregnancy, may well be the treatment of the future, alongside more established advice such as giving up smoking and cutting down on alcohol.'

In addition, certain people are not genetically predisposed to tolerate certain foods in their diets. Coeliac disease, for example, is much more common among the Irish, Finnish, Sardinians and possibly Native Americans.

Don't abuse alcohol

Drinking alcohol can increase anyone's allergy risk because it makes the gut more leaky by irritating the digestive tract. Research conducted by the University of Western Australia's Asthma and Allergy Research Institute has identified that wine in particular can trigger asthma attacks. They found that among 366 asthma sufferers, 1 in 3 reported that alcoholic drink triggered asthma attacks. Such reports were more common from people using steroid drugs or inhalers. In wine, the allergens involved may be sulphites,[103] while yeast or salicylates may also play a part.

Cross-reactions – when sensitivities link

Another contributor to food sensitivity is exposure to allergens drifting around in the atmosphere. For example, it is well known that when the pollen count is high, more people suffer from hay fever in polluted areas than in rural areas, despite the lower pollen counts in cities. Exposure to exhaust fumes is thought to make a pollen-allergic person more sensitive. Whether this is simply because their immune system is weakened from dealing with the pollution and therefore less able to cope with the additional pollen insult, or due to some kind of 'cross-reaction', is not known. In the US, where ragweed sensitivity is common, a cross-reaction with bananas has been reported. In other words, one sensitivity sensitises you to another. Hay-fever sufferers may develop cross-reactions involving pollen, wheat and milk.

The emerging view, shared by an increasing number of allergy specialists, is that food sensitivity is a multi-factorial phenomenon possibly involving poor nutrition, pollution, digestive problems and overexposure to certain foods. Removing the foods may help the immune system to recover, but other factors need to be dealt with for any major impact on long-term food allergy to be made.

Addiction to problem foods

One interesting finding among people with food allergies is that they often become hooked on the very food that causes a reaction. This can actually lead to bingeing on the foods that harm them most. Many people describe these foods as making them feel drugged or dopey. In some cases, the foods induce a mild state of euphoria. For these people, the food in question can actually become a psychological escape mechanism and a way of dealing with uncomfortable situations. But why do some foods cause drug-like reactions?

When pain no longer serves a purpose as part of a survival mechanism, chemicals called endorphins are released. These are the body's natural painkillers, and they make you feel good. The way they do this is by binding to sites that turn off pain and turn on pleasant sensations. Opiates such as morphine are similar in chemical structure and bind to the same sites, which is why they suppress pain.

Endorphins, whether made by the body or taken as a drug, are peptides – small groups of amino acids bound together. When a protein you eat is digested, it first becomes peptides and then, if the digestion works well, single amino acids. In the laboratory, endorphin-like peptides have been made from wheat, milk, barley and corn using human digestive enzymes. These peptides have been shown to bind to endorphin receptor sites. Preliminary research does seem to show that certain foods, most commonly wheat and milk, may induce a short-term positive feeling, even if, in the long term, they are causing health problems. In autistic children, milk and gluten endorphin-like chemicals are usually found in the urine, indicating leaky gut problems.

So it seems that frequently, the foods that don't suit you are also the foods you 'couldn't live without'. And in the first few days of giving up a suspect food, you may in fact start feeling pretty rough before you feel better. Some things are addictive in their own right: sugar, alcohol, coffee, chocolate and tea (especially Earl Grey, which also contains the addictive essential oil, bergamot). You can react to these foods without being allergic. Wheat and milk could be added to this list on the basis of their endorphin-like effects.

■ Reversing IgG food allergies

Now you know all the factors that minimise your chances of developing allergies. Some you can act on now. Others, such as whether you were breast-fed or have a genetic legacy to deal with, are beyond your control. But the real trick to reversing your allergic tendency and losing your IgG allergies lies in two golden rules:

- Strictly avoid what you are allergic to
- Heal your gut.

Simply avoid it

What location is to a property that is for sale, strict elimination of allergic foods is to treating food allergy. Eliminating allergic foods means exactly that. Find out what you are allergic to by having an IgG food allergy test then strictly avoid your allergy foods for three to six months. This will demand very careful reading of labels on cans and packages, and exercising caution in restaurants.

The reason for the 3 to 6 months is that the IgG antibodies have a 'half-life' of 6 weeks. This means that after 6 weeks, half of your IgG antibodies have died and been replaced, and after 12 weeks another half have died and been replaced. After 3 to 6 months you no longer have any of the IgG antibodies you had to start with. Provided you've been avoiding the foods you're allergic to, the new IgG antibodies inside you will no longer react to your food allergen if you reintroduce it.

This does not apply to IgE-based, immediate-onset food allergies or to coeliac disease. As far as we know, the only cure is lifelong avoidance of the food, although the anti-allergy diet and supplements we recommend will reduce your degree of allergic sensitivity.

Heal the gut

There are several possible underlying reasons why a person becomes food allergic. We've investigated a number of them: a lack of digestive enzymes, leaky gut, frequent exposure to foods containing irritant chemicals, immune deficiency leading to hypersensitivity of the immune system, and no doubt many more. Fortunately, tests exist to identify deficiencies in digestive enzymes, leaky gut syndrome, and the balance of bacteria and yeast in the gut. They can be arranged through nutritionists. To find one in your area, please see Resources on page 170.

There is a lot you can do to allow the gut and immune system to calm down and your allergic potential to decrease:

- Take digestive enzyme complexes (lipase, amylase and protease) that help digest fat, protein and carbohydrate. Since stomach acid and protein-digesting enzymes rely on zinc and vitamin B6, it may help to take 15mg of zinc and 50mg of B6 twice a day, as well as the digestive enzyme with each meal.

- Help heal your leaky gut. Cell membranes are made out of fat-like compounds, and one fatty acid – butyric acid – helps to heal the gut wall. The ideal daily dose is 1,200mg. Vitamin A is also crucial for the health of any mucous membrane, including the gut wall, and taking 5g of powdered glutamine (an amino acid) in water before bed is also an excellent aid in helping the gut heal.

- Beneficial bacteria such as *Lactobacillus acidophilus* or *Bifidobacteria* can also help to calm down a reactive digestive tract.

- Boosting your immune system reduces any hypersensitivity it may have developed. Antioxidant nutrients and foods, vitamin A, B vitamins, zinc and selenium all help to do this.

We look more closely at the foods, herbs and nutrients that will help you fight food allergy below. And in Chapter 8, we put it all together: we'll tell you exactly what to eat and what to supplement in our 30-day digestive healing regime.

Anti-allergy foods, herbs and nutrients

There are specific anti-allergy and anti-inflammatory foods, nutrients and herbs that help to calm a hyped-up immune system. Let's take a look at these because each one is a vital piece of your action plan for food allergy relief, explained in Chapter 8.

Cornucopia of health – fruit and veg

The more fresh fruit and vegetables you eat, the lower your risk of allergy. Specifically, apples, kiwi fruit and oranges have all been shown to reduce the incidence of asthma symptoms.[104–105] Apples are especially high in quercetin (more on this anti-allergy phytonutrient later).

Both fruit and vegetables are high in antioxidant nutrients

that help calm down allergic reactions. Among these, vitamin C is probably the most powerful, and one we recommend you also supplement (see Chapter 8). Onions and garlic contain the sulphur-rich amino acids cysteine and methionine, which help reduce allergic potential. It's also better to eat organic – not only because you do actually get more of these nutrients in organic produce, but also because that way you don't get exposed to a wide variety of toxic chemicals that can induce allergy in their own right.

The essential fats – omega-3s

The last three decades have seen a dramatic increase in the prevalence of asthma, eczema, otitis media, ADHD, allergic rhinitis and many other allergy-related conditions. In parallel with this increase in allergy, there has been a decrease in the amounts of omega-3 fatty acids we are getting in our diets. Omega-3s are essential fatty acids found most abundantly in oily fish and flaxseeds (also called linseeds). A true superfood, they protect our cells, promote brain health, balance our hormones and reduce inflammation – which is why they're important in treating allergies.

But many are failing to get the message. Along with the decline in omega-3 consumption there has been an upswing in the amount of vegetable and seed oils (omega-6 fatty acids) – in margarine, for instance – we're eating. The vegetable oils used in processed foods are especially bad news because the omega-6 fats they contain become damaged, and promote inflammation in the body. The imbalance caused by eating more omega-6s than omega-3s is unhealthy, too, as it can lead to overproduction of chemical troublemakers called inflammatory prostaglandins and leukotrienes, which make you more prone to chronic inflammation and allergies.[106]

In a study published in the *Medical Journal of Australia*, children who regularly ate fresh, oily fish had a significantly reduced risk of and protection from asthma. No other food groups or nutrients were associated with either an increased or reduced risk.[107] This is thought to be because a diet with a high omega-3 to omega-6 ratio makes you less likely to produce IgE antibodies and become allergic.[108] So by eating more fresh, oily fish and other sources of omega-3 oils, you can reduce your allergic potential.

Flaxseeds and their oil are an excellent omega-3 option, particularly for vegetarians. The ancient Greek physician and 'father of medicine' Hippocrates wrote of using flaxseed for the relief of abdominal pain. And the greatest of all medieval kings, Charlemagne, considered flaxseed so healthy that he passed laws requiring its consumption. Along with its high omega-3 content, flaxseed is also very rich in fibre and lignans. Lignans are phytoestrogens (plant substances that mimic the action of the hormone oestrogen) that are thought to bind to oestrogen receptors in the body, and may have a role in preventing hormonally related cancers of the breast, uterus lining and prostate gland. Although lignans are found in most unrefined grains (barley, buckwheat, millet and oats), soya beans and some vegetables (broccoli, carrots, cauliflower and spinach), flaxseed is the richest source.

Flaxseed contains both soluble and insoluble fibre (about 28g total fibre per 100g of flaxseed). About a third of the fibre is soluble. Studies have found that the soluble fibre in flaxseed – like that found in oat bran and fruit pectin – can help lower cholesterol and regulate blood sugar. The remaining two-thirds of the fibre in flaxseed is insoluble, which aids digestion by increasing bulk, reducing the time that waste remains in the body and preventing constipation.

Incorporating flaxseed into a diet is simple and can add a tasty twist to routine foods and dishes. The small, reddish-brown whole seeds have a nutty taste and can be sprinkled over salads, soups, yoghurt or cereals; grinding them will make the omega-3s more available. Whole or ground flaxseed can replace some of the flour in bread, muffin, pancake and biscuit recipes. Flaxseed oil is also readily available in health food stores and may be substituted for other oils; ensure you keep it in the fridge to prevent it from going rancid.

So it makes good food allergy-fighting sense to eat grilled or poached (never fried or breaded) wild or organic salmon, trout, mackerel, sardines, herring or other oily fish, accompanied by a bountiful mixed salad dressed with cold-pressed flaxseed oil. If you're vegetarian, go for walnuts, pumpkin seeds, sesame seeds and omega-3 enriched eggs in addition to flaxseeds.

MSM – the magic molecule

MSM (methylsulfonylmethane) is a non-toxic, natural component of the plants and animals we eat and is also normally found in breast milk. This magic molecule contains a highly usable form of sulphur, the fourth most abundant mineral in the human body and part of the chemical make-up of over 150 compounds (all the proteins, as well as sulphur-containing amino acids, antibodies, collagen, skin, nails, insulin, growth hormone and the most potent antioxidant, the enzyme glutathione). Vegans and people on a high-carbohydrate, low-protein diet probably don't get enough MSM. Antibiotic overuse may also contribute to sulphur deficiency by killing off the intestinal bacteria needed to produce essential sulphur-containing amino acids.

Correcting a deficiency is important, as MSM has a number of proven benefits:

- It alleviates allergic responses to food and pollen allergens. The anti-allergic property of MSM is reported to be on a par with or better than traditional antihistaminic drugs.

- It provides relief for migraine headache sufferers.

- Daily supplementation is reported to provide dramatic and long-lasting relief of rheumatoid arthritis pain.

- It helps prevent and reverse the constipation seen in people with IBS and cow's milk allergy.

- It helps relieve snoring, a common food allergy symptom.

- Acne, acne rosacea, and diverse other skin problems associated with a leaky gut and food allergy respond favourably to MSM supplementation.

- It is particularly helpful for people experiencing allergy-related pain, stiffness and swelling.

MSM appears to relieve allergies in a number of ways. It binds to or coats the lining of the small intestine, which may help soothe inflammation and reverse a leaky gut. MSM also provides the intestinal bacteria with building blocks for the manufacture of major anti-allergy, anti-inflammatory sulphur-containing amino acids, such as methionine and cysteine. Cysteine goes on to increase the production of glutathione, low levels of which are associated with an increased risk of premature death from all causes.

MSM is as safe as drinking water, and the daily therapeutic dose ranges from 1,000 to 6,000mg. It works better if taken with vitamin C. Bear in mind that MSM is not like an aspirin or a shot of cortisol. A single, one-time dose of it is rarely effective in lessening symptoms. Reduction in pain, inflammation and other allergic symptoms are usually seen within 2 to 21 days.

Glutamine – fuelling immunity

L-glutamine is an amino acid, literally the most abundant in the human body. It is the most important food or fuel for the small intestinal mucosa and the immune system. Like the MSM-derived amino acid, cysteine, glutamine is critical in maintaining optimal levels of the detoxifying, life-protecting antioxidant enzyme glutathione.

When in ample supply – that is, when you're well and not overly stressed from food allergies, coeliac disease, Crohn's disease, ulcerative colitis or chronic inflammation, or recovering from a major injury or excessive exercise – glutamine is able to quickly heal an inflamed intestine and maintain a healthy intestinal lining and immune system. If, on the other hand, you are chronically stressed from food allergy, leaky gut and a suppressed immune system, you will also be suffering from glutamine deficiency and will benefit from glutamine supplementation.

Taking glutamine has proven therapeutic benefits:

- It increases glutathione production in the liver, lymph nodes, intestinal lining, brain and airways. This helps the food-allergy sufferer clear immune complexes (see page 22) from circulation.

- It helps prevent and reverse leaky gut, including coeliac disease, Crohn's disease, and ulcerative colitis.

- It helps prevent intestinal bleeding and ulceration in patients taking aspirin and other non-steroidal anti-inflammatory drugs (NSAIDs) for food allergy-induced chronic pain syndromes such as arthritis, migraines and fibromyalgia. In Japan, patients taking NSAIDs for pain and inflammation are instructed to take 2g of L-glutamine 30 minutes beforehand to prevent stomach bleeding and ulceration.

- It helps prevent or reverse poor nutrient status in food allergy patients experiencing malabsorption of nutrients.

- It helps prevent and heal peptic ulcers, a condition worsened by food allergy.

To get the best results with glutamine, you'll need to take 4g of glutamine powder – roughly one heaped teaspoon – dissolved in an 8oz glass of water, two or three times a day.

Anti-allergy antioxidants

Aside from their general role in keeping you optimally nourished, a number of key vitamins and minerals will help reduce your allergic potential.

Vitamin A is an extremely important antioxidant and immune system-enhancing vitamin. Signs of deficiency include mouth ulcers, poor night vision and skin problems such as acne. Here are some of its allergy-busting functions in the body:

- It maintains health of the mucous membranes and skin.

Helpful in the prevention and treatment of eczema, psoriasis and acne.

- As an antioxidant, it disarms highly destructive molecules, or free radicals, released during allergic reactions.

- It maintains a healthy thymus gland, the master gland of the immune system.

- It helps prevent the release of excessive inflammatory prostaglandins during allergic reactions.

- Along with zinc and probiotics, it helps in the production of two substances playing an important role in the digestive tract – protective mucus, and secretory IgA, which prevents bacteria, yeast, parasites and food allergens from contacting the intestinal lining and passing into the bloodstream.

Vitamin A is of therapeutic value in the treatment of asthma, IBS, eczema, rheumatoid arthritis and other food allergy-related disorders. Except for women who have not reached the menopause, a basic dose of 6,000mcg a day is very safe for most adults, and 3,000mcg is minimal. Premenopausal women should not take more than 1,500mcg of vitamin A a day because too much of this vitamin is associated with a potentially increased risk of birth defects. Also, as with all fat-soluble vitamins, there is the possibility of toxicity from overdoses of vitamin A.

Your individual tolerance level will depend on your metabolism, and general state of health. Signs that you are taking too much vitamin A can be dry skin, irritability, tenderness or aching in the long bones of the body, headaches, cracking at the edges of the lips, hair thinning or loss, and abnormal liver function tests. Stop taking it to relieve the symptoms. Recognising the possible side effects of vitamin A supplementation, however, should not scare you away from including substantial amounts of this vital anti-allergy supplement in your daily regime.

Vitamin B6, in addition to being a major antioxidant, plays a big part in the metabolism of essential fatty acids into prostaglandins, and therefore has far-reaching effects on the cardiovascular, digestive, neurological and immune systems. This vitamin is also linked to learning, behavioural, emotional and mental processes, and plays a critical co-factor role in the production of serotonin, a neurotransmitter that seems to play an important role in alleviating food allergy-induced chronic pain, headaches and depression. Signs of a deficiency include tingling in the hands, depression, premenstrual symptoms and low energy levels.

Vitamin B6 affects food allergies in a number of ways:

- It improves the production and release of hydrochloric acid in the stomach. Food allergy sufferers often don't produce enough stomach acid, probably because of food allergy-induced gut hormone inhibition and malnutrition. B6 works better when taken in conjunction with niacin (B3), zinc and a diet that eliminates food allergens.

- It helps relieve food allergy or gluten-induced psychological depression and ADHD-related hyperactivity.

- It helps in the treatment of certain forms of epilepsy and chronic pain syndromes.

- It stimulates the thymus gland, thereby contributing to the formation of antibodies and more optimally functioning immune cells.

B6 deficiency is one of the most common nutrient deficiencies, yet the RDA for this vitamin is pitifully low – just 2mg a day. Many top nutritional scientists believe that a more optimal proper intake should be at least ten times this amount – 20mg. There are no safety concern regarding amounts up to 200mg.

Vitamin C is a natural antihistamine, enhancing the action of the enzyme histaminase, which quickly breaks down histamine. That means it will give you instant relief during a histamine-based allergic reaction such as hay fever, as long as you take enough. One gram of vitamin C reduces blood histamine by approximately 20 per cent, and 2g reduces histamine by over 30 per cent.[109]

But there's much, much more to this phenomenal vitamin. C seems to be involved in almost all bodily functions. It is needed for the replacement of old tissue and the generation of new, making it invaluable for the healing of inflamed tissues and wounds. Healthy teeth and bones depend on its presence for strength and flexibility, as do the walls of capillaries and veins.

The vitamin's most profound effects, however, are in its overall strengthening of the immune system. It stimulates certain white blood cells, the phagocytes, to seek out and devour food allergens, bacteria and viruses.

Vitamin C also acts as a powerful antioxidant, detoxifying many harmful free radicals, both in the environment and in the body, where the molecules can be produced during allergic reactions. C is also known to reactivate vitamin E, another powerful antioxidant. Asthmatics, especially those suffering from exercise-induced asthma, as well as hay fever sufferers and people with food-induced allergic rhinitis or arthritis, can benefit from the immune support provided by vitamin C.

If you're short on C, you may have bleeding gums, bruise easily and catch frequent colds and infections.

How much C should you take? The minimum maintenance dose is 500mg a day. The adult therapeutic dose begins at about 2,000mg a day. As much as 8,000 to 12,000mg daily, in divided doses, such as 1g every two hours, may be indicated if you're having a severe allergic reaction; however, this is for short-term use only. The only reported side effect, even with these large amounts, is loose bowels.

It's a myth that vitamin C causes kidney stones. People with calcium oxalate kidney stones, which account for about 80 per cent of all kidney stones, often lack magnesium and B6. Supplementing these can help prevent calcium oxalate kidney stone formation.

Magnesium is the second most abundant mineral in the human body. It works closely with calcium and vitamin B6 to regulate the heart, muscles, brain and immune system. Research has shown that magnesium has a calming effect, working as a natural sedative – hence it's sometimes called the 'anti-stress mineral'.

Magnesium is also needed for essential fats to work properly, and plays a significant role in the prevention and treatment of various allergy-related conditions such as premenstrual syndrome, asthma, hyperactivity, autism and migraine. During migraine attacks, an intravenous administration of 1g of magnesium has been shown to reverse the attack in over 80 per cent of cases.[110–111] Magnesium supplements also help reduce symptoms of asthma, and intravenous magnesium at the time of an asthma attack has been shown to halve recovery time. If you're not getting enough, you may experience constipation, cramps, headaches, insomnia and depression.

We recommend taking 200mg of elemental magnesium as a

chelate (such as magnesium glycinate, citrate or ascorbate) two to three times daily.

Zinc has turned out to be far more influential in the treatment of food allergy than anyone thought. The mineral is a vital co-factor of essential fatty acid metabolism. Along with niacin and B6, it is important for the production of hydrochloric acid in the stomach.

Zinc is a powerful immune-system stimulant.[112] It activates the thymus gland, which in turn produces the immune cell-stimulating hormone thymosin. Zinc is known to aid in restoring the delicate linings of the airways, and healing the gastrointestinal tract – in short, reversing a leaky gut. It also increases the levels of secretory immunoglobulin A (IgA) in the saliva and gut. (Secretory IgA protects the gut by preventing bacteria, yeast, parasites and food allergens from contacting the lining and passing into the bloodstream.) And it is needed for IgG antibody production.

Warning signs of a zinc deficiency include coeliac disease, chronic inflammatory skin conditions, wounds that don't heal, poor dark light adaptation, poor appetite, anorexia nervosa, retarded growth in a child, abnormal cravings for carbohydrates and sweets, impaired taste or smell, and frequent recurring infections.

Although the RDA for zinc is 15mg per day, doses of 20 to 40mg have had beneficial effects in conditions common among food allergy sufferers, such as acne, dermatitis herpetiformis (an extremely itchy rash associated with coeliac disease), eczema, psoriasis, hyperactivity, eating disorders and learning disabilities. Daily doses of 40mg or higher should not be continued for longer than three months. Zinc depletes the body of copper. Therefore, it is recommended that 1mg of copper should also be supplemented with every 10 to 15mg of zinc.

Quercetin The one daily supplement that often reduces allergic symptoms across the board is quercetin, a chemical compound known as a bioflavonoid and found in plants. Sometimes, using just quercetin, a person can reintroduce allergen foods with no symptoms.

Quercetin is naturally found in wine, but not beer; tea, but not coffee; and the outer layers of red and yellow onions, but not white onions. Apples, lettuce, chives, berries, cherries, algae, tree bark and other plant materials also contain quercetin. The most studied, potent and versatile of all 4,000 or so bioflavonoids, quercetin stabilises mast cells in allergic patients. These mast cells, as we've seen, are unstable in allergy sufferers, and too readily release large quantities of histamine, inflammatory prostaglandins, cytokines, leukotrienes, and others of the chemical culprits behind allergic symptoms. Quercetin is also a potent antioxidant and anti-inflammatory agent.

For the best effect, quercetin should be taken in combination with vitamin C and a high-potency bromelain, the enzyme found in pineapple. For most people, the effective therapeutic dose is 500mg of quercetin in combination with approximately 125mg of high-potency bromelain and 250 to 500mg vitamin C, taken 30 minutes before meals, 2 to 3 times a day. For maintenance (after your allergic symptoms have been brought under good control), reduce the above dose to once or twice daily, 30 minutes before breakfast and/or again before dinner.

Now we're ready to show you how to build all these and other anti-allergy foods, herbs and nutrients into a powerful action plan for food allergy relief, using diet and supplements. We show you the ropes in the next chapter, including what to do for immediate relief if you have an allergic reaction.

8

Your Action Plan for Food Allergy Relief

IN THIS CHAPTER we'll show you the most effective way to overcome your allergies by giving you the maximum chance of 'unlearning' some of them, and minimising any reactions you do have.

It's important to note, however, that these techniques won't work if you have coeliac disease, or immediate-onset allergies to foods like peanuts or shellfish, involving serious allergic reactions such as asthma or anaphylaxis. (We are assuming, by this stage, that you have found what you are allergic to by having an IgG food allergy test, a coeliac screening test and possibly an IgE food allergy test too.) As far as we know, an immediate-onset IgE allergy means a permanent, fixed food hypersensitivity, and you must carefully avoid the allergen all your life.

However, in most cases, you can reverse – and even lose – delayed-onset IgG food allergies. Here's how you do it.

■ 1. Eliminate your food allergens

There's no way round it: to treat an IgG food allergy, you need to start by strictly eliminating the allergen, and then rotating it with non-allergens (more on this soon). This means that for three to six months, you need to avoid that food – no ifs, ands or buts.

For now, think in terms of three months minimum. You'll need to think beyond the obvious – read all the labels on tins and packets, question waiters in restaurants, anything to be sure of avoiding that particular food. If it's a favourite of yours, you'll need to be willing to give it up, and perhaps go through a few withdrawal or detoxification symptoms over a few days. This may make you feel deprived – as if you miss a 'good friend' who can temporarily make you feel better. But remember: it also means the end of allergic suffering and freedom from nagging, chronic, disabling physical, mental and emotional symptoms. There's a good chance that you'll be feeling so fantastic at the end of our three-month programme, you simply won't miss your allergic foods.

However, you'll need to be realistic from the start. Expect mild-to-moderate withdrawal or detoxification symptoms when coming off your allergens. Physiological addiction to food is no different from addiction to alcohol, caffeine or tobacco. If you have allergies of a fairly severe nature, you can expect to go through a withdrawal period that usually lasts three to five days. The withdrawal symptoms usually reflect an intensification of symptoms you were already having, including headache, fatigue, poor sleep, anxiety, depression, irritability, stuffiness, joint aches, digestive upset and severe food cravings. (One extremely effective treatment that helps prevent severe withdrawal is supplementing with large, therapeutic doses of vitamin C. Take 1g every other hour, up to a maximum of 12g in one day, and continue for three consecutive days. If you get diarrhoea during this time, halve the amount you take.)

■ 2. Eats lots of fruit and vegetables

As we learnt in Chapter 7, eating lots of fruit and vegetables actually reduces your allergic potential, and gives you a great supply of antioxidants and other important nutrients. Whenever you can, eat organic, especially for foods you eat raw and unpeeled such as apples, pears, berries, tomatoes and raw carrots. Make sure you always have a big bowl full of delicious fruit and veg for you and your family to snack on. Have something raw with most meals.

Many fruits and vegetables are also high in the anti-allergy nutrient quercetin. This not only acts as an anti-inflammatory, calming down any reactions that you have. It also calms down the immune system's mast cells (which release allergy-causing chemicals such as histamine), thereby reducing your allergic potential.

As you'll see from the chart opposite, the best vegetables for quercetin are, by a long way, red onions, followed by spinach, carrots and broccoli. The best commonly available fruits to go for are apples and berries, especially cranberries and blueberries (red grapes are high in glucose, which can have a disruptive effect on blood sugar balance). We recommend you aim for at least 10mg a day, although the more you take in from your diet the better. The chart above shows you what that means in terms of what you eat. If you are a coffee drinker, think of changing to quercetin-rich tea.

Food	Quercetin (mg) per 100 g food
Red onions	19.93
Cranberries	14.02
Spinach	4.86
Apples	4.42
Red grapes	3.54
Carrots	3.50
Broccoli	3.21
Blueberries	3.11
Lettuce	2.47
Sweet cherries	1.25
Plums	1.20
Blackberries	1.03
Raspberries	0.83
Green peppers	0.65
Strawberries	0.65
Tomatoes	0.57
Pears	0.42

▪ 3. Go fish

By now we've seen how a diet high in omega-3 fish oils reduces your allergic tendency. While a small number of people are allergic to white fish, few are allergic to the oily fish such as salmon, mackerel, herring, sardines and tuna, which are the best source of omega-3 fats. Basically, fish that eat fish tend to be highest in omega-3. There are also other nutrients found in fish, in addition to the oils, that may prove helpful in preventing and relieving many of the symptoms of food allergy. They include selenium, sterols and NADH, a substance synthesised from niacin (vitamin B3) that's contained in all living cells. However, very large fish like swordfish and tuna can have substantial amounts of mercury in them, as this accumulates too. So eat wild or organic salmon or smaller oily fish as much as possible, aiming for three times a week.

■ 4. Easy on grains and dairy

Enough has been said and proven about the dangers of a diet high in dairy and gluten, or at least gliadin grains. So, go easy on wheat in particular and vary your diet so it isn't dependent on grains every day. Eat non-gliadin oats, and non-gluten grains such as buckwheat, rice, quinoa, corn and millet. Vary your diet as much as possible.

■ 5. Rotate your foods

Working out a new pattern to your eating so you're not consuming the same foods every day is – after avoiding allergens, healing a leaky gut and the rest – the single most important thing you can do to reverse and prevent a recurrence of food allergy.

Most food allergy tests will identify the foods you need to avoid (because they cause a significant antibody reaction) and foods that you can rotate (because they cause very little or no antibody reaction). If your allergy test doesn't specify foods to rotate, you can apply this principle to everything you eat, and certainly any of the foods in the top 20 food allergens listed in Chapter 5. In practice, what rotating will mean is that you will only eat that food once every three to four days – and preferably, less frequently.

So for at least the first three months following the complete elimination of all your food allergens, carefully rotate either those your food allergy test or health professional has advised you to rotate or, if you don't have this information, the top 20 food allergens. Rotating foods in this way really takes a load off your immune system and increases your chances of being able to reintroduce most of your allergens back into your daily diet – without allergic symptoms.

After three months, the principles of food rotation should still guide what and how you eat, though on a much more flexible basis. Nevertheless the principles of rotation are the foundation of an allergy-free life. Here's why:

1 A rotation diet helps prevent the development of allergies and thus addictions. Food allergies develop for a wide variety of reasons, but a major one seems to be too frequent and/or too large an exposure to a potential food allergen, especially in the context of a leaky gut. (Our Stone Age ancestors, who had the same genetic make-up as us, were forced by seasons and scarcity to rotate and vary their foods).

2 Rotation encourages a more balanced, unprocessed and varied diet and therefore leads to consuming more needed nutrients. If you are not going to repeat foods more often than every three days, you will have to get out of your eating rut! Most people's diets are dominated, calorie-wise, by no more than ten foods and beverages, ingested almost every day of their lives.

3 Rotation dictates a simple, unrefined, additive-free diet. It is almost impossible to continue to eat processed, packaged foods on a rotation diet. Many packaged foods contain not 1 or 2, but dozens of food ingredients, which, once eaten, cannot be eaten again for 72 to 96 hours. The same goes for recipes with multiple ingredients and elaborate sauces or gravies.

4 Rotation unstresses digestion. A rotation diet is what your digestive system was genetically designed to handle. Without overexposure to the same foods, food allergens, 'bad' fats and oil, chemicals, additives and excess refined sugar, your system can quickly strengthen and repair itself. Varied, nutrient- and fibre-rich, non-allergic foods bring about the optimal release of gut hormones and digestive juices; help heal and reverse an inflamed, leaky gut lining; improve absorption of nutrients; reduce toxic overload to the liver; and relieve constipation and diarrhoea.

5 Food allergen-free rotation often leads to dramatic weight loss – often without calorie counting or restriction of calories. A rotation diet clears up the allergies that lead to food cravings, overeating, a slowed metabolism and water retention.

To plan a rotation diet, begin with a list of the foods to which you are not allergic. The next step is to plan three to four days of menus. Again, the meal plans should avoid all the foods to which you are allergic and should not repeat any non-allergic food for 3 or 4 days.

In this planning process, be guided by what you like, the time you have to prepare meals, and what is available at local supermarkets or health food stores. Keep it simple: use just a few foods and ingredients in each meal. If you have to avoid protein-rich foods like eggs, beef and dairy products, make sure you get protein from alternative sources – non-allergenic fresh poached, baked or grilled fish, or lentils and beans, for example. Here are some additional tips to make your rotation diet a success:

1 Be an alert shopper. Some common allergic foods show up in dozens of popular food items. That is why it is best to eat simple, fresh foods as much as possible.

2 Avoid all alcohol, or keep it to an absolute minimum, for three months (booze of any kind is a major cause of a leaky gut).

3 Have a big, fresh, mixed vegetable salad every day; not eating enough fresh vegetables each day is a fundamental cause of allergy. The choice of salad dressing is important. Rotate your oils daily and select only unrefined, cold-pressed oils. Our preferences include cold-pressed flaxseed oil and extra virgin olive oil.

4 Drink eight glasses of bottled or filtered water or herbal teas each day.

5 Try not to eat after 7 pm and make the last meal of the day a lighter meal. Allow at least two hours between the end of your meal and bedtime.

6 There is no limit, except satisfaction of physiological hunger, on the amount that you eat. Do not count calories, do not remain hungry and do not starve yourself.

Concentrate on good nutrition and your health. If you're overweight, you'll be amazed when your weight begins to plummet without self-denial, and without counting a single calorie.

Food families also need to be considered when you plan your rotation diet, since it is possible for a cross-reaction to occur to close relatives of foods you have an intolerance for. Foods from any one food family (see Appendix 1) should be eaten on the same day and, where possible, not eaten again for the next three days.

For example, if your food allergy test advises you to rotate cow's milk, rice, wheat, pea, salmon, pork, soya beans and yeast, here's an example of how to do it, with the food family shown in (*italics*).

DAY 1	DAY 2	DAY 3	DAY 4
Wheat (*grass*)	Salmon	Pea (*legume*)	Pork
Rice (*grass*)	Yeast	Soya (*legume*)	Cow's milk

■ How to reintroduce foods

Anyone who finds they have food allergies inevitably will ask the question, 'Will I ever be able to eat the food(s) again?' After eliminating allergy-provoking foods for at least three months, and preferably six, most people with delayed food allergies find they can 'clear' most of their food allergies. If done cautiously, one food at a time, you will be able reintroduce most of your formerly allergic foods back into your diet without allergic symptoms. Then, the chances are you will remain allergy-free, provided you continue to avoid the mistakes and bad dietary choices that led to food allergy in the first place.

On the other hand, life is not always fair. As we've said, people with coeliac disease (gluten allergy) or with severe IgE allergies to peanuts or shellfish and symptoms such as anaphylaxis, asthma or severe angioedema will have to carry syringes of adrenalin and anti-histamine medication with them at all times. Needless to say, their respective allergens must also be carefully avoided for a lifetime.

Otherwise, here's how you go about reintroducing a food. After three months of strict rotation, reintroduce a moderate serving of a previously offending foods back into your diet, one food at a time, every three days. If you're still allergic to certain foods, the three days allows time for delayed food allergic reactions to occur.

Depending on your allergies, here are the best foods for you to reintroduce, and guidelines to make the reintroduction of foods most effective:

- If dairy has been avoided then a plain 'bio-live' yoghurt is the best to test first. If no reactions occur over a five-day period, try cow's milk.

- If wheat has been avoided, try a wheat-only product such as shredded wheat. Likewise, with oats, make a porridge of oats with water so it is only the oats themselves you are testing. The same is advisable with other grains.

- Egg is best tested by trying the cooked yolk only. If there is no reaction within five days then egg white could be tested next.

- When testing any of the foods choose a food made only of

the product to be tested so you are positive it contains no other products.

- Always allow one week between reintroducing new foods. Any reaction and symptoms need to be monitored over the testing period.

- Reintroduce foods in ascending order of the severity of the reaction as given in your test results. So that means starting with the foods that gave the weakest reaction because your body is more likely to have forgotten about these foods first.

To make it easy for you, we've included a symptom score chart in Appendix 2 for you to use to record your symptoms as you reintroduce foods. In this way you can keep a clear record of what happens. If you do not react in three days, then it is likely that you can reintroduce this food into your diet, although we advise that you continue to rotate it and/or eat the food infrequently.

■ Anti-allergy Supplements

In addition to eliminating your food allergens and following a rotation diet, certain natural supplements can help you to recover more quickly from food allergies and decrease your allergic potential. We had a look at these in the previous chapter – now let's see how you put it into action.

Immune-boosting Supplements

Your immune system depends on a minute-by-minute supply of a wide range of nutrients, especially vitamin A, B vitamins, zinc, magnesium and selenium. In addition to eating a nutrient-rich, non-allergic whole food diet we recommend that you supplement these nutrients on a daily basis.

Here's the kind of levels you want to supplement on a daily basis:

Vitamin A	1,500mcg
Beta-carotene	500mcg
Vitamin B6	20mg
Magnesium	200mg
Zinc	15mg

You can find all of these in a good high-strength multivitamin. The best multivitamin and mineral supplements recommend taking two a day, for the simple reason that you can't get all these ideal levels into one tablet or capsule.

Even so, you'll never find enough vitamin C in a multi, so this needs to be taken separately as well. We recommend anyone with allergies to supplement 1,000mg twice a day and possibly more, especially if you are in the withdrawal phase or still experiencing allergic symptoms.

Anti-allergy and anti-inflammatory supplements

Vitamin C is the most important anti-allergy vitamin. It is a powerful promoter of a strong immune system, immediately calms down allergic reactions and is also anti-inflammatory. It's really recommended for everyone at an absolute minimum of 1,000mg (1g) a day, although 2,000mg (2g) or more is optimum for most people, whether or not you have allergies. If you are suffering from allergic symptoms, you might want to take twice this amount on a regular basis. Since vitamin C is in and out of the body within six hours, it's best taken in divided doses, either 1g in the morning and 1g at lunch or, if you're taking larger amounts, 1g four times a day. (Note: if you have a history of recurring kidney stones, it is advisable that you take extra vitamin B6 and magnesium, in a decent multivitamin for example, daily with your vitamin C.)

Omega-3 fish oils are one of nature's best natural anti-inflammatory nutrients, with countless other benefits besides. Although you can and should obtain these from eating unfried, unbreaded fish, we recommend you supplement omega-3 fish oils every day as an insurance policy. To give you a rough idea, we recommend you take in the equivalent of 1,000mg of combined EPA and DHA (these are the two most powerful omega-3 fatty acids) a day, or 7,000mg a week. A 100g serving of mackerel might give you 2,000mg, while a serving of salmon might give you 1,000mg. So, if you eat fish three times a week you'll probably achieve 3,500mg a week. To make up the remaining 3,500mg we recommend you take an omega-3 fish oil supplement providing 500mg of combined EPA and DHA a day. This is good advice for anyone, even if you're not especially allergic.

Quercetin, like omega-3 and vitamin C, is provided in the foods we recommend you eat, but you'll be hard pushed to eat more than 20mg a day. That's good and to be highly recommended, but supplementing 500mg three times a day when suffering from severe allergies and 500mg a day once you have your allergies under control as a maintenance dose is effective for reducing allergic potential. The best results are achieved by supplementing 250mg, twice a day, with some bromelain (digestive enzyme from pineapple) and vitamin C. Some quercetin supplements contain all these in one.

MSM has so many benefits for allergy sufferers that it's hard to know where to start. As long as you're still suffering from any allergic symptoms, or in pain, it's well worth supplementing MSM on a daily basis. While therapeutic intakes go up to 6,000mg a day, we recommend you start with 1,000mg twice a day.

Glutamine is an essential part of any regime designed to quickly restore a healthy digestive tract and prevent further damage from foods, alcohol or medications. It is also a powerful nutrient for supporting proper immune function and protecting the liver. For this reason, we not only recommend it as part of healing a leaky gut, but also for anyone during the first 30 days of following an action plan for food allergy relief. The ideal amount is 8 to 16g mixed and consumed in cold or warm (not hot) water each day. A heaped teaspoon is about 4g. So two heaped teaspoons a day is recommended. For best results drink the glutamine solution on an empty stomach, on waking and before bed.

Each of these five nutrients is non-toxic and we highly recommend you take them for the first 30 days to rapidly reduce your allergic potential. If you find them particularly effective and wish to continue supplementing them on a regular basis, go ahead – you'll be doing your overall health a massive favour.

■ Your prescription for healing the gut

Allergies and leaky gut syndrome is one of those chicken-or-egg situations. There's good reason to suppose that having a more permeable digestive tract is what precipitates food allergies in the first place, while having a food allergy encourages a leaky gut by inflaming the digestive tract wall. While you can test for increased gastrointestinal permeability, it's highly likely that you have a degree of increased permeability, especially if you have multiple food allergies or digestive symptoms. Since the digestive tract lining is rapidly replacing itself, here's what you can do in 30 days to quickly improve the health of your inner skin, thereby reducing your allergic potential. These recommendations complement the diet and supplement action points discussed above, rather than replacing them:

Digestive enzymes that help digest fat, protein and carbohydrate – that is, lipase, amylase and protease – are well worth trying if you have any digestive problems or food allergy symptoms. Since stomach acid and protein-digesting enzymes rely on zinc and vitamin B6, it may help to take 15mg of zinc and 50mg of B6 twice a day, as well as a digestive enzyme with each meal.

Butyric acid or caprylic acid are medium-chain triglycerides (blood fats) and help to heal the gut wall, partly because the membranes of intestinal cells are largely made out of such fats. The ideal daily dose of either is 900mg to 1,200mg a day, or 300mg to 400mg three times a day.

Probiotics such as *Lactobacillus acidophilus* or *Bifidobacteria* can also help to calm down a reactive digestive tract and reduce allergic potential. Probiotic bacteria need to eat to survive. This is where 'prebiotics' come into play. Prebiotics are non-digestible, fermentable food ingredients that feed and stimulate friendly bacteria in the intestines. They increase the densities of beneficial bacteria and stimulate growth and functions of the healthy intestine. Recent findings show that after acute diarrhoea, giving a prebiotic accelerates recovery of beneficial bacteria, reduces the relative abundance of detrimental, disease-causing bacteria, stimulates intestinal mucosal growth and enhances digestion and immunity.[115] Prebiotics are often included in probiotic supplements for this reason. Examples of prebiotics include fructooligosaccharides (FOS), inulin (from fermentable chicory fructan, a kind of carbohydrate), guar gum and pectin. Look out for probiotic supplements containing these as well as a billion or more viable organisms, providing both *Lactobacillus* and *Bifidobacteria*.

The action plan: a recap

In short, here's what to do to minimise your allergic potential and swiftly become allergy-free.

Your anti-allergy diet

- Eliminate your food allergens
- Follow a three- or four-day rotation diet
- Minimise wheat and milk products even if you're not allergic
- Have a large mixed salad every day and at least three portions of vegetables
- Have at least three pieces of fruit every day
- Eat at least 10mg of quercetin each day from foods such as red onions, apples and berries, although you'll benefit from more in supplements
- Eat unfried, unbreaded oily fish rich in omega-3 fats – such as mackerel, sardines or wild or organic salmon – three times a week
- Eat ground flaxseeds and pumpkin seeds, and use flaxseed oil in salad dressings
- Drink eight glasses of water or herbal teas every day.

▶

Your anti-allergy supplements

	AM	PM
Every day		
■ High-strength multivitamin	1	1
■ Vitamin C 1,000mg	1	1
■ Omega-3 fish oils (500mg of EPA/DHA)	1	
For the first 30 days (otherwise optional)		
■ Quercetin 500mg+	1	1
■ MSM 1,000mg	1	1
■ Glutamine powder* (1 teaspoon = 4g)	1 tsp	1tsp
Additional nutrients for healing a leaky gut		
■ Digestive enzymes	1 with each meal	
■ Probiotics (*Lactobacillus*, *Bifidobacteria*) plus prebiotics such as FOS	1 with each meal	
■ Butyric acid or caprylic acid 350mg	1 with each meal	

Unless otherwise stated, take nutritional supplements with food. Glutamine powder is best taken in water on an empty stomach, first thing in the morning and/or last thing at night. Occasionally, some people find glutamine too energising if taken last thing at night.

See Resources for a directory of supplement companies.

PS: What to do if you've had an allergic reaction

If you are having an allergic reaction and want to recover as quickly as possible, here's what to do until the allergic symptoms subside:

- Stop eating!

- Drink only filtered water and drink plenty of it (at least ten glasses of water during the day). A measure that you are drinking enough is that you'll have to urinate frequently, and that the urine will be clear.

- Begin taking large therapeutic doses of crystal vitamin C (as ascorbic acid) = one rounded teaspoon of vitamin C (about 2 to 4g) every 30 to 60 minutes until it causes watery stools – not loose stools, but diarrhoea. This may take 8 to 24 hours.

- Then, reduce to 1/2 teaspoon every hour until the symptoms are gone. (Note: If you have a history of recurring kidney stones, you should also be taking 400mg of magnesium and 50mg of vitamin B6 daily during this time).

- When your allergic symptoms are gone and you begin eating again, be extremely careful to avoid all the foods you were eating during the three days before the onset of your allergic reaction. And eat much smaller portions of all foods for several days. Otherwise, you may react again!

Appendix 1

Know Your Food Families

AS THEY'RE ALL based on plants or animals, foods can be grouped into families depending on which ones they're derived from, and will share similar proteins with their close relatives. It's well worth knowing these food families. For example, both cashew nuts and pistachios are from the *cashew* family. This means that if you react to one, you are more likely to react to the other. *Crustaceans* – crab, crayfish, lobster, prawn and shrimp – are quite different from *molluscs*, which include abalone, clams, cockles, mussels, oysters, scallops, snails and squid. Octopus is in a family of its own. If you react to crustaceans, there is no reason why you should react to *mollusc* or *octopus* family foods.

FAMILY NAME	FOODS IN THE FAMILY

Plants

Banana	Banana, plantain, ginger, turmeric, arrowroot, vanilla
Beech	Beechnut, chestnut
Beet	Beet, chard, spinach, sugar beet
Berry	Blackberry, boysenberry, loganberry, raspberry, strawberry
Birch	Hazelnut, wintergreen
Buckwheat	Buckwheat, rhubarb, sorrel
Carrot	Angelica, caraway, carrot, celery, chervil, coriander, cumin, dill, fennel, parsley, parsnip
Cashew	Cashew nuts, mango, pistachio
Citrus	Citron, grapefruit, lemon, lime, mandarin, orange, tangerine
Composites	Artichoke, chamomile, chicory, dandelion, endive, lettuce, safflower, sunflower, salsify, tarragon
Fungi	Mushrooms, truffle, yeast
Gourd	Courgette, cucumber, gherkin, melon (honeydew), pumpkin, squash, watermelon
Grape	Grape, raisin, sultana, cream of tartar (a byproduct of winemaking)
Grass	Bamboo shoots, barley, corn, millet, oat, rice, rye, sugar cane, sorghum, wheat
Heather	Blueberry
Laurel	Avocado, bay leaf, cinnamon, sassafras
Lily	Asparagus, chive, garlic, leek, onion, shallot
Legume	Bean, lentil, liquorice, pea, peanut, senna, soya, tapioca, carob
Madder	Coffee
Mint	Basil, bergamot, lavender, lemon balm, marjoram, mint, oregano, rosemary, sage, thyme

Mulberry	Breadfruit, fig, hop, mulberry
Mustard	Broccoli, Brussels sprouts, cabbage, Chinese leaves, cauliflower, cress, horseradish, kale, kohlrabi, mustard, radish, rapeseed, turnip, watercress
Olive	Olive
Palm	Coconut, date, palm, sago
Pineapple	Pineapple
Potato (nightshade family)	Aubergine (eggplant), paprika, pepper, cayenne pepper, chilli pepper, potato, sesame, tahini, tobacco, tomato
Rose	Apple (including cider), crab apple, pear, rosehip
Rosestone family	Almond, apricot, cherry, nectarine, peach, plum, prune, quince, sloe
Saxifrage	Blackcurrant, currant, gooseberry
Stericula	Chocolate, cocoa, cola
Tea	Tea
Verbena	Lemon verbena
Walnut	Butternut, pecan nut, walnut

Poultry and wildfowl

Dove	Pigeon
Duck	Duck, goose
Grouse	Grouse, partridge
Guinea fowl	Guinea fowl
Pheasant	Chicken (and their eggs), peafowl, pheasant, quail
Turkey	Turkey

Meat

Bovid	Beef, buffalo, veal, beef dairy products (cow's milk, cream, whey, yoghurt, cheese), gelatine, goat, goat's milk and cheese, lamb, sheep's milk and cheese, feta, Roquefort

Deer	Caribou, elk, moose, reindeer, venison
Hare	Hare, rabbit
Swine	Pork

Seafood

Crustacean	Crab, crayfish, lobster, prawn, shrimp
Mollusc	Abalone, clam, cockle, mussel, oyster, scallop, snail, squid
Octopus	Octopus

Freshwater fish

Bass	Bass, perch (white), yellow bass
Herring	Shad
Minnow	Carp, chub
Perch	Perch (yellow), red snapper
Pike	Pickerel, pike
Salmon	Salmon, trout
Smelt	Smelt
Sturgeon	Caviar, sturgeon
Sunfish	Black bass

Saltwater fish

Anchovy	Anchovy
Codfish	Cod, cod liver oil, haddock, hake, pollock
Eel	Eel
Flounder	Flounder, halibut, plaice, sole, turbot
Sea herring	Herring, sardine, pilchard
Mackerel	Mackerel, tuna, bonito
Mullet	Mullet
Porgy	Bream, porgy
Salmon	Salmon, sea trout
Scorpion fish	Ocean perch, rockfish

Sea bass	Grouper, sea bass
Sea catfish	Catfish
Skate	Skate

| **Honey** | Honey contains multiple plant pollens, while commercial honey frequently contains sugar |

FOOD FAMILIES BY INDIVIDUAL FOODS

Food Item	Family	Food Item	Family
Grains			
Barley	*Grass*	Buckwheat	*Buckwheat*
Corn (maize)	*Grass*	Malt	*Grass*
Millet	*Grass*	Oat	*Grass*
Rice	*Grass*	Rye	*Grass*
Sago	*Palm*	Tapioca	*Grass*
Wheat	*Grass*		
Dairy			
Brie	*Bovid*	Cheddar	*Bovid*
Cottage cheese	*Bovid*	Edam	*Bovid*
Egg (whole)	*Pheasant*	Evaporated milk	*Bovid*
Goat's cheese	*Bovid*	Goat's milk	*Bovid*
Gouda	*Bovid*	Cow's milk	*Bovid*
Processed cheese	*Bovid*	Sheep's milk	*Bovid*
Stilton	*Bovid*	Swiss cheese	*Bovid*
Whey (cow's)	*Bovid*	Yoghurt	*Bovid*

Food Item	Family	Food Item	Family
Meat/poultry			
Beef	*Bovid*	Chicken	*Pheasant*
Duck	*Duck*	Lamb	*Bovid*
Liver (beef)	*Bovid*	Pork	*Swine*
Rabbit	*Hare*	Turkey	*Turkey*
Venison	*Deer*		
Fish			
Anchovy	*Anchovy*	Clam	*Mollusc*
Cod	*Codfish*	Crab	*Crustacean*
Haddock	*Codfish*	Halibut	*Flounder*
Mackerel	*Mackerel*	Mussels	*Mollusc*
Oyster	*Mollusc*	Pilchard	*Sea herring*
Plaice	*Flounder*	Prawn	*Crustacean*
Salmon	*Salmon*	Sardine	*Sea herring*
Scallop	*Mollusc*	Skate	*Skate*
Sole	*Flounder*	Trout	*Salmon*
Tuna	*Mackerel*		
Vegetables			
Artichoke (eggplant)	*Composite*	Asparagus	*Lily*
Aubergine	*Potato*	Avocado	*Laurel*
Butterbeans	*Legume*	Kidney beans	*Legume*
Beansprouts	*Legume*	Beetroot	*Beet*
Broccoli	*Mustard*	Cabbage	*Mustard*
Carob	*Legume*	Cauliflower	*Mustard*
Carrot	*Carrot*	Chickpea	*Legume*
Celery	*Carrot*	Cucumber	*Gourd*
Courgette (zucchini)	*Gourd*	Green beans	*Legume*
Endive	*Composite*	Leek	*Lily*

Food Item	Family	Food Item	Family
Haricot beans	*Legume*	Lettuce	*Composite*
Lentils	*Legume*	Onion	*Lily*
Parsnip	*Carrot*	Pea	*Legume*
Potato	*Potato*	Pinto beans	*Legume*
Radish	*Mustard*	Potato (sweet)	*Morning glory*
Safflower	*Composite*	Rhubarb	*Buckwheat*
Spinach	*Beet*	Soya bean	*Legume*
Squash	*Gourd*	Sprouts (Brussels)	*Mustard*
Tomato	*Potato*	Sunflower	*Composite*
Turnip	*Yam*	Mustard	*Yam*

Fruits

Food Item	Family	Food Item	Family
Apple	*Rose*	Apricot	*Rosestone*
Banana	*Banana*	Blackberry	*Berry*
Blackcurrant	*Saxifrage*	Blueberry	*Heather*
Cherry	*Rosestone*	Date	*Palm*
Fig	*Mulberry*	Gooseberry	*Saxifrage*
Grape	*Grape*	Grapefruit	*Citrus*
Hops	*Mulberry*	Kiwi	*Kiwi*
Lemon	*Citrus*	Lime	*Citrus*
Mango	*Cashew*	Melon	*Gourd*
Olive	*Olive*	Orange	*Citrus*
Peach	*Rosestone*	Pear	*Rose*
Pineapple	*Pineapple*	Plum	*Rosestone*
Raspberry	*Berry*	Strawberry	*Berry*
Sultana	*Grape*		

Food Item	Family	Food Item	Family
Nuts			
Almond	*Rosestone*	Brazil nut	*Brazil*
Cashew nut	*Cashew*	Chestnut	*Beech*
Coconut	*Palm*	Hazelnut	*Birch*
Peanut	*Legume*	Pecan nut	*Walnut*
Pistachio	*Cashew*	Walnut	*Walnut*
Spices/herbs			
Arrowroot	*Banana*	Basil	*Mint*
Bay leaf	*Laurel*	Cayenne pepper	*Potato*
Chicory	*Composite*	Chilli	*Potato*
Cinnamon	*Laurel*	Coriander	*Carrot*
Fennel	*Carrot*	Garlic	*Lily*
Ginger	*Banana*	Liquorice	*Legume*
Mustard	*Mustard*	Nutmeg	*Nutmeg*
Oregano	*Mint*	Sesame seed	*Potato*
Parsley	*Carrot*	Pepper (black)	*Peppercorn*
Pepper (white)	*Peppercorn*	Rosemary	*Mint*
Sage	*Mint*	Sesame seed	*Potato*
Tarragon	*Composite*	Thyme	*Mint*
Tobacco	*Potato*	Turmeric	*Banana*
Vanilla	*Banana*		
Others			
Beet sugar	*Beet*	Chamomile	*Composite*
Cane sugar	*Grass*	Chocolate/cocoa	*Stericula*
Coffee	*Madder*	Cola	*Stericula*
Maple syrup	*Maple*	Mushrooms	*Fungi*
Rape seed	*Mustard*	Tea	*Tea*
Yeast	*Fungi*		

Appendix 2

Symptom Score Chart

THE CHART BELOW is designed for people with IgG delayed-onset allergies who have cut their allergen foods out for three months (see page 131) and want to reintroduce those foods. If that's you, this chart will help you monitor that process.

We recommend that you keep a daily record of what you eat, any symptoms that you might be having, and any other factor that might alter your progress. It is also advisable to keep a record of your weight, since weight gain is a frequent symptom of food allergy.

Note that we've devised a scoring system that you may find helpful when you're trying to gauge how each symptom is affecting you each day.

The scores are as follow: 3 = very bad
2 = bad
1 = not too bad/improving
0 = not a problem

	Day/date	Symptoms and Score	Weight	Notes
1				1st avoid food reintroduced
2				
3				
4				
5				
6				
7				
8				2nd avoid food reintroduced
9				
10				
11				
12				
13				
14				
15				3rd avoid food reintroduced
16				
17				
18				
19				
20				
21				

	Day/date	Symptoms and Score	Weight	Notes
22				4th avoid food reintroduced
23				
24				
25				
26				
27				
28				
29				5th avoid food reintroduced
30				
31				
32				
33				
34				
35				
36				6th avoid food reintroduced
37				
38				
39				
40				
41				
42				

	Day/date	Symptoms and Score	Weight	Notes
43				7th avoid food reintroduced
44				
45				
46				
47				
48				
49				
50				

Appendix 3

Coeliac Disease

COELIAC DISEASE IS A permanent, serious condition characterised by an allergic toxicity to gliadin – a glycoprotein (carbohydrate plus protein) found in gluten cereals. If people with this illness consume any gliadin (and it doesn't take much – less than half a gram), the gliadin will attack the lining of their intestines. The lining becomes leaky and loses its ability to absorb nutrients from food. Malabsorption and malnutrition set in, along with deficiencies in iron, zinc, calcium, magnesium, potassium and vitamins B6, B12, folic acid, A, D, E and K.

There is a strong genetic aspect to coeliac disease. Seventy per cent of identical twins both get it, making it 175 times more prevalent than in the general population – which points to a probable genetic tendency. If you have a mother, father, brother or sister with coeliac disease, you have a 1 in 10 chance of having it too – or in other words, a 30 times higher risk than the average person.

Medical textbooks still say that it occurs in only 1 in 5,000 or so people. Due to remarkable advances in laboratory screening for coeliac sufferers, we have learnt that it occurs more frequently than anyone ever imagined. According to a random sampling by the American Red Cross, 1 in 250 people in the US suffer from coeliac disease – and 19 out of every 20 cases go undetected and untreated. More recent studies appearing in the top medical journal the *Lancet* have reported a prevalence of 1 in 122 Irish, 1 in 85 Finnish, 1 in 70 of Italians in northern Sardinia,[113] and 1 in 18 Algerian Saharawi refugee children.

Coeliac disease is thought to be such a health threat in Italy that the government has considered mandating that all children, regardless if they are sick or not, must be tested for gliadin sensitivity and coeliac disease by the age of six. In Britain we are still in the Dark Ages in terms of recognising the widespread prevalence of coeliac disease.

■ A shift in signs and symptoms

The other medical myth about coeliac disease is that a doctor should be able to diagnose a patient easily through 'unmistakable' abdominal and other signs and symptoms: chronic diarrhoea/episodic diarrhoea with malnutrition, abdominal cramping, abdominal distention or bloating, foul-smelling, bulky stools (steatorrhoea), weight loss or poor weight gain, short stature, and a patient complaining of weakness, fatigue and loss of appetite.

This scenario is changing irrevocably, however. Today, most people with undiagnosed coeliac disease no longer go to the doctor complaining of abdominal problems. Instead, they could come through the door with a whole range of varied symptoms:

- Chronic psychological depression

- Overweight or obesity

- Abnormal elevation of liver enzymes of unknown cause

- Permanent teeth with distinctive horizontal grooves and chalky whiteness

- Chronic nerve disease of unknown cause (such as ataxia or peripheral neuropathy)

- Osteoporosis in women not responding to conventional therapies

- Intestinal cancers

- Insulin-dependent diabetes

- Thyroid disease (both overactive and underactive)

- Short stature in children.

Undetected gluten sensitivity, whether or not it has led to coeliac disease, is commonly found among pre- and post-menopausal women and even children who suffer from osteoporosis. The same nutrient deficiencies found in osteoporosis – magnesium, vitamin D and vitamin K – are also seen in people suffering from coeliac disease. In fact, one recent study showed that a gluten-free diet actually reversed osteoporosis in people with coeliac disease. They took 44 coeliac patients aged from 2 to 20 at the time of their diagnosis, and compared them with 177 healthy, coeliac-free people. The lumbar spine and whole-body bone mineral density values of people with coeliac disease were significantly lower than those of people without it. After a year and a half on a gluten-free diet, the people with coeliac disease were retested and it was found that their bone density had improved to the point where it was almost indistinguishable from that of the non-coeliacs.[114]

Undetected coeliac disease is associated with a forty- to hundredfold increased risk of intestinal lymphomas[115] – cancers of the lymphatic system. This is because the immune system of a person with coeliac disease doesn't fight cancer cells as well as it should. Over 80 international studies have been published on the increased incidence of cancer in people with this disease. In the case of intestinal lymphomas, once these have reached the point where they are diagnosed, the prognosis is generally very poor. But the good news is this: if coeliac disease is diagnosed before these intestinal lymphomas become evident, and a gluten-free diet is strictly followed, the risk of developing this cancer decreases from a hundredfold back to near normal in just five years.

The prevention of cancer is the single most compelling argument for routine and repeated screening or monitoring for coeliac disease in people with any of the above conditions, symptoms or a close relative with the disease.

▪ The only known cure

The only known effective therapy for coeliac disease is the complete, life-long elimination of gluten from the diet. No wheat, rye or barley in *any* form is allowed. Initially, we also recommend avoiding oats – but if an IgG food allergy test does not show the presence of oat antibodies, you could try reintroducing oats. About 80 per cent of coeliac disease sufferers can tolerate oats.

If strictly followed, this regime swiftly and dramatically brings the sufferer back to health. Diseased intestines heal; deficient nutrients are again absorbed; bones get stronger; the high risk of intestinal cancer returns to a normal one (see above). But you have to suspect and diagnose coeliac disease first!

Given that, it's wonderful that there has been a revolution in laboratory testing and screening for coeliac disease. Hopefully, if these new tests are used intelligently, often – and soon – by health professionals, better health for the tens of millions of gluten-sensitive people round the world will be swiftly on its way.

References

1. Royal College of Physicians special report, *Containing the Allergy Epidemic* (June 2003)
2. *US News and World Report*, vol 106, pp 77 (1989)
3. Dixon, H, Treatment of delayed food allergy based on specific immunoglobulin G RAST testing, *Otolaryngol Head Neck Surgery*, vol 1213, pp 48–54; and independent scientific audit of 2,567 patients with long-term illnesses by the Department of Health Studies at the University of York, UK, on behalf of the British Allergy Foundation. Study and fact sheet published 22 January 2001
4. Zuberbier, T *et al.*, Department of Dermatology, Virchow-Klinikum, Humboldt University, Berlin, Germany, Pseudoallergen-free [food additive free] diet in the treatment of chronic urticaria, *Acta Derm Ventereol*, vol 75, pp 484–487 (1995)
5. McDonald P J *et al.*, Food protein-induced enterocolitis: Altered antibody response to ingested antigen, *Pediatr Res*, vol 18, pp 751–5 (1984)
6. Lindberg E *et al.*, Antibody (IgG, IgA, and IgM) to baker's yeast (*Saccharomyces cerevisiae*), yeast mannan, gliadin, ovalbumin and betalac-toglobulin in monozygotic twins with inflammatory bowel disease, *Gut*, vol 33, pp 909–13 (1992)

7. Snook, J and Shepherd, H A, Bran supplementation in the treatment of irritable bowel syndrome, *Aliment Pharmacol Ther,* vol 8, pp 511–514 (1994)

8. Francis, C Y and Whorwell, P J, Bran and irritable bowel syndrome: Time for reappraisal, *Lancet,* vol 344, pp 39–40 (1994))

9. Atkinson, W *et al.,* Do food elimination diets improve Irritable Bowel Syndrome? A double blind trial based on IgG antibodies to food, *Gut,* vol 53, pp 1391–1393 (2004)

10. Sameer, Z *et al.,* Food-specific serum IgG4 and IgE titers to common food antigens in irritable bowel syndrome, *Am J of Gastroenterol,* vol 100, pp 1550–1557 (2005)

11. Sameer, Z *et al.,* Food-specific serum IgG4 and IgE titers to common food antigens in irritable bowel syndrome, *Am J of Gastroenterol,* vol 100, pp 1550–1557 (2005)

12. Wahnschaffe, U *et al.,* Disease-like intestinal antibody pattern in patients with irritable bowel syndrome (IBS), *Gastroenterology,* vol 114, pp A430 (1998)

13. Wahnschaffe, U *et al.,* Celiac disease-like abnormalities in a subgroup of patients with irritable bowel syndrome, *Gastroenterology,* vol 121, pp 1329–38 (2001)

14. Straus, S E *et al.,* Allergy and the chronic fatigue syndrome, *J Allergy Clin Immunol,* vol 81 pp 791–795 (1988)

15. Baraniuk, J N *et al.,* Rhinitis symptoms in chronic fatigue syndrome, *Ann Allergy Asthma Immunol,* vol 81, pp 359–365 (1998)

16. van den Bergh, V *et al.,* Trigger factors in migraine, *Headache,* vol 27, pp 191–195 (1987)

17. Egger, J *et al.,* Is migraine food allergy? A double-blind placebo-controlled trial of oligoantigenic diet treatment, *Lancet,* vol 2, 865–869 (1983)

18. Hughes, E *et al.,* Migraine: A diagnostic test for etiology of food sensitivity by a nutritionally supported fast and confirmed by long term report, *Ann Allergy,* vol 55, pp 28–33 (1985)

19. Mansfield, L *et al.,* Food allergy and adult migraine: Double-blind and mediator conformation of an allergic etiology, *Ann Allergy,* vol 55, pp 126–129 (1985)

20. van der Laar, M A and van der Korst, J K, Food intolerance in rheumatoid arthritis I: A double blind, controlled trial of the clinical effects of elimination of milk allergens and azo dyes, *Ann Rheum Dis,* vol 51, pp 298–302 (1992); van der Laar, M A and van der Korst, J K, Food intolerance in rheumatoid arthritis II: Clinical and histological aspects, *Ann Rheum Dis,* vol 51, pp 303–306 (1992)

21. Firer, M A *et al.*, Cow's milk allergy and eczema: Patterns of the antibody response to cow's milk in allergic skin disease, *Clin Allergy*, vol 12, pp 385–90 (1982)

22. Shakib, F *et al.*, Relevance of milk- and egg-specific IgG4 in atopic eczema, *Int Arch Allergy Appl* Immunol, vol 75, pp 107–12 (1984); Shakib F *et al.*, Study of IgG sub-class antibodies in patients with milk intolerance, *Clin Allergy*, vol 16, pp 451–8 (1986)

23. Husby, S *et al.*, IgG subclass antibodies to dietary antigens in atopic dermatitis, *Acta Derm Venereol Suppl*, vol 144, pp 88–92 (1989)

24. Iikura, Y *et al.*, How to prevent allergic disease I. Study of specific IgE, IgG, and IgG4 antibodies in serum of pregnant mothers, cord blood, and infants, *Int Arch Allergy Appl Immunol*, vol 88, pp 250–2 (1989)

25. Lucarelli, S *et al.*, Specific IgG and IgA antibodies and related subclasses in the diagnosis of gastrointestinal disorders or atopic dermatitis due to cow's milk and egg, *Int J Immunopathol Pharmacol*, vol 11, pp 77–85 (1998)

26. Niggemann, B *et al.*,, Outcome of double-blind, placebo-controlled food challenge tests in 107 children with atopic dermatitis, *Clin Exp Allergy*, vol 29, pp 91–96 (1999)

27. Boushey, H *et al.*, Daily versus as-needed corticosteroids for mild persistent asthma, *N Engl J Med. Apr* 14, 352, pp 1589–91 (2005)

28. Sicherer, S H, Leurg, D Y, Advances in allergic skin disease, anaphylaxis, and hypersensitivity reactions to food, drugs, and insects, *J Allergy Clin Immunol*, vol 116, pp 153–63 (2005). Kanny, G, Atopic dermatitis in children and food allergy: combination or causality?, *Ann Dematol Venereol*, 132 Spec No. 1, 1590–103 (2005)

29. Danesch U C, Petasites hybridus (butterbur root) extract in the treatment of asthma – an open trial, *Altern Med Rev*, vol 9, pp 54–62 (2004)

30. Randolph, T, Allergy as a causative factor of fatigue, irritability and behaviour problems of children, *J Pediatr*, vol 31, pp 560 (1947)

31. Rowe, A, Allergic toxemia and fatigue, *Ann Allergy*, vol 17, pp 9 (1959)

32. Speer, G, Allergy of the Nervous System, Thomas (1970)

33. Campbell, M, Neurologic manifestations of allergic disease, *Ann Allergy*, vol 31, pp 485 (1973)

34. Hall, K, Allergy of the nervous system: A review, *Ann Allergy*, vol 36, pp 49–64 (1976)

35. Pippere, V, Some varieties of food intolerance in psychiatric patients, *Nutr Health*, vol 3, pp 125–136 (1984)

36. Pfeiffer, C and Holford, P, *Mental Illness and Schizophrenia: The Nutrition Connection*, Thorsons (1989)

37. Tuormaa, T, *An Alternative to Psychiatry*, The Book Guild (1991)

38. Vlissides D *et al.*, A double-blind gluten-free/gluten-load controlled trial in a secure word population, *British Journal of Psychiatry*, vol 148, pp 447–52 (1986)

39. Jyonouchi H *et al.*, Dysregulated innate immune responses in young children with autism spectrum disorders: their relationship to gastro-intestinal symptoms and dietary intervention, *Neuropsychobiology*, vol 51, pp 77–85 (2005)

40. Egger, *et al.*, Controlled trial of oligoantigenic diet treatment in the hyperkinetic syndrome, *Lancet*, vol 1, pp 540–545 (1985)

41. Feingold, B, Dietary management of behaviour and learning disabilities, in *Nutrition and Behavior*, S.A. Miller (ed), Franklin Institute Press (1981), p 37

42. Egger, J *et al.* (1985)

43. Carter, C M *et al.*, Effects of a few food diet in attention deficit disorder, *Arch Dis Child*, vol 69, pp 564–8 (1993)

44. Whiteley, P, Sunderland University Autism Unit, presentation to 'Autism Unravelled' conference, London, May 2001

45. Rosenfeld, R M, What to expect from medical treatment of otitis media, *Pediatr Infect Dis J*, vol 14, pp 731–738 (1995)

46. Van den Broek, P *et al.*, Letter to the editor, *Lancet*, vol 348, pp 1517 (1996)

47. Williams, R L *et al.*, Use of antibiotics in preventing recurrent acute otitis media and in treating otitis media with effusion, *JAMA*, vol 270, pp 1344–1351 (1993)

48. Soutar, A, Bronchial reactivity and dietary antioxidants, *Thorax*, vol 52, pp 166–170 (1997)

49. Rebuffat, E *et al.*, Difficulty in initiating and maintaining sleep associated with cow's milk allergy in infants, *Sleep*, vol 10, pp 116–121 (1987)

50. Kahn, A *et al.*, Milk intolerance in children with persistent sleeplessness: A prospective double-blind crossover evaluation, *Pediatrics*, vol 84, pp 595–603 (1989)

51. Robson, W L *et al.*, Enuresis in children with attention-deficit hyperactivity disorder, *SC South Med J*, vol 90, pp 503–5 (1997)

52. Egger, J, *et al.*, Effect of diet treatment on enuresis in children with migraine or hyperkinetic behavior, *Clin Pediatr (Phila)*, vol 31, pp 302–307 (1992)

53. Scott, F W *et al.*, Potential mechanisms by which certain foods promote or inhibit the development of spontaneous diabetes in BB rats: Dose, timing, early effect on islet area, and switch in infiltrate from Th1 to Th2 cells, *Diabetes*, vol 46, pp 589–598 (1997)

54. Lorini, R *et al.*, Clinical aspects of coeliac disease in children with insulin-dependent diabetes mellitus, *J Pediatr Endocrinol Metab*, Suppl 1, pp 101–111 (1996)

55. Sjöberg, K *et al.*, Screening for coeliac disease in adult insulin-dependent diabetes mellitus, *J Intern Med*, vol 243, pp 133–40 (1998)

56. Holmes, G K *et al.*, Coeliac disease and Type 1 diabetes mellitus: The case for screening, *Diabet Med*, vol 18, pp 69–77 (2001)

57. Mohn A, *et al.*, Celiac disease in children and adolescents with type I diabetes: Importance of hypoglycemia, *Pediatr Gastroenterol Nutr*, vol 32, pp 37–40 (2001)

58. Not, T *et al.*, Undiagnosed celiac disease and risk of autoimmune disorders in subjects with type I diabetes, *Diabetologia*, vol 44, pp 151–5 (2001)

59. Kumar, V *et al.*, Celiac disease-associated autoimmune endocrinopathies, *Diagn Lab Immunol*, vol 8, pp 678–85 (2001)

60. Ventura, A *et al.*, Gluten-dependent diabetes-related and thyroid-related autoantibodies in patients with celiac disease, *J Pediatr*, vol 137, pp 263–265 (2000)

61. Toscano, V *et al.*, Importance of gluten in the induction of endocrine autoantibodies and organ dysfunction in adolescent celiac patients, *Am J Gastroenterol*, vol 95, pp 1742–1748 (2000)

62. Kitts, D *et al.*, Adverse reactions to food constituents: Allergy, intolerance, and autoimmunity, *Can J Physiol Pharmacol*, vol 75, pp 241–54 (1997)

63. *The Immunology Review*, vol 2 (1994)

64. Cohen G A *et al.*, Severe anemia and chronic bronchitis associated with a markedly elevated specific IgG to cow's milk protein, *Ann Allergy*, vol 55, pp 38–40 (1985)

65. Fallstrom, S P *et al.*, Serum antibodies against native, processed and digested cow's milk proteins in children with cow's milk protein intolerance, *Clin Allergy*, vol 16, pp 417–23 (1986)

66. Shakib, F *et al.*, Study of IgG sub-class antibodies in patients with milk intolerance, *Clin Allergy*, vol 16, pp 451–8 (1986)

67. Host, A *et al.*, Prospective estimation of IgG, IgG subclass and IgE antibodies to dietary proteins in infants with cow's milk allergy. Levels of antibodies to whole milk protein, BLG and ovalbumin in relation to repeated milk challenge and clinical course of cow's milk allergy, *Allergy*, vol 47, pp 218–29 (1992)

68. Hamburger, R N *et al.*, Long-term studies in prevention of food allergy: Patterns of IgG anti-cow's milk antibody responses, *Ann Allergy*, vol 59, pp 175–8 (1987)

69. Taylor, C J *et al.*, Detection of cow's milk protein intolerance by an enzyme-linked immunosorbent assay, *Acta Paediatr Scand*, vol 77, pp 49–54 (1988)

70. Iacono, G *et al.* IgG anti-beta lactoglubolin (beta lactotest): its usefulness in the diagnosis of cow's milk allergy, *It J Gastroentol*, vol 27, pp 355–360 (1995)

71. Cavataio, F *et al.*, Gastroesophageal reflux associated with cow's milk allergy in infants: Which diagnostic examinations are useful?, *Am J Gastroenterol*, vol 91, pp 1215–20 (1996)

72. Duchateau, J *et al.*, Anti-betalactoglobulin IgG antibodies bind to a specific profile of epitopes when patients are allergic to cow's milk proteins, *Clin Exp Allergy*, vol 28, pp 824–33 (1998)

73. US National Institutes of Health (http://digestive.niddk.nih.gov/ddiseases/pubs/lactoseintolerance/)

74. Feskanich, D *et al.*, Milk, dietary calcium, and bone fractures in women: A 12–year prospective study, *Am J Public Health*, vol 87, pp 992 (1997)

75. Paspati, I. *et al.*, Hip fracture epidemiology in Greece during 1977–1992, *Calcif Tissue Int*, vol 62, pp 542–547 (1998)

76. Lau, E M and Cooper, C, Epidemiology and prevention of osteoporosis in urbanized Asian populations, *Osteoporosis*, vol 3, pp. 23–26 (1993)

77. Fujita, T and Fukase, M, Comparison of osteoporosis and calcium intake between Japan and the United States, *Proc Soc Exp Biol Med*, vol 200, pp 149–152 (1992)

78. Xu, L *et al.*, Very low rates of hip fracture in Beijing, People's Republic of China: The Beijing Osteoprosis Project, *Am J Epedemiol*, vol 144, pp 901–907 (1996)

79. Torgerson, J *et al.*, Randomised controlled trial of calcium and supplementation with cholecalciferol (vitamin D3) for prevention of fractures in primary care, *BMJ*, vol 330, pp 1003 (2005)

80. Gerarduzzi, T *et al.*, Celiac disease in USA among risk groups and general population in USA, *J Pediatr Gastroenterol Nutr*, vol 31, pp 104 (2000)

81. Sandiford, CP *et al.*, Identification of the major water/salt insoluble wheat proteins involved in cereal hypersensitivity, *Clin Exp Allergy*, vol 27, pp 1120–1129 (1997)

82. Högberg, L *et al.*, Oats to children with newly diagnosed coeliac disease: A randomised double blind study, *Gut*, vol 53, pp 649–654 (2004)

83. Størsrud, S *et al.*, Adult coeliac patients do tolerate large amounts of oats, *Eur J Clin Nutr*, vol 57, pp 163–169 (2003)

84. Cooke, S K and Sampson, H A, Allergenic properties of ovomucoid in man, *J Immunol*, vol 159, pp 2026–2032 (1997)

85. Lever, R et al., Randomised controlled trial of advice on an egg exclusion diet in young children with atopic eczema and sensitivity to eggs, *Pediatr Allergy Immunol*, vol 9, pp 13–9 (1998)

86. Rance, F and Dutau, G, Labial food challenge in children with food allergy, *Pediatr Allergy Immunol*, vol 8, pp 41–44 (1997)

87. Urisu, A et al., Allergenic activity of heated and ovomucoid-depleted egg white, *J Allergy Clin Immunol*, vol 100, pp 171–176 (1997)

88. Saxena, I and Tayyab, S, Protein proteinase inhibitors from avian egg whites, *Cell Mol Life Sci*, vol 53, pp 13–23 (1997)

89. Atkinson W et al., Food elimination based on IgG antibodies in irritable bowel syndrome: a randomised controlled trial, vol 53, pp 1459–64 (2004)

90. Sblattero, D et al., Human recombinant tissue transglutaminase ELISA: An innovative diagnostic assay for celiac disease, *Am J Gastroenterol*, vol 95, pp 1253–1257 (2000)

91. Jalonen, T, Identical permeability changes in children with different clinical manifestations of cow's milk allergy, *J Allergy Clin Immunol*, vol 88, pp 737–742 (1991)

92. Wagner, R D et al., Biotherapeutic effects of probiotic bacteria on candidiasis in immunodeficient mice, *Infect Immun*, vol 65, pp 4165–4172 (1997)

93. Matsuzaki, T and Chin, J, Modulating immune responses with probiotic bacteria, *Immunol Cell Biol*, vol 78, pp 67–73 (2000)

94. Majamaa, H and Isolauri, E, Probiotics: A novel approach in the management of food allergy, *J Allergy Clin Immunol*, vol 99, pp 179–185 (1997)

95. Zheng, T et al., Lactation reduces breast cancer risk in Shandong Province, China, *Am J Epidemiol*, vol 152, pp 1129–1135 (2000)

96. Tomkins, A, Malnutrition, morbidity and mortality in children and their mothers, *Proc Nutr Soc*, vol 59, pp 135–146 (2000)

97. Hoppu, U et al., Maternal diet rich in saturated fat during breastfeeding is associated with atopic sensitization of the infant, *Eur J Clin Nutr*, vol 54, pp 702–705 (2000)

98. Dandrifosse, G et al., Are milk polyamines preventive agents against food allergy? *Proc Nutr Soc*, vol 59, pp 81–6 (2000)

99. Jensen-Jarolim, E, research presented at World Allergy Organization's (WAO) Congress in Vancouver, Canada, 6–12 September 2003

100. Johnson, C et al., Antibiotic exposure in early infancy and risk for childhood atopy, *J Allergy Clin Immunol*, vol 115, pp 1218–1224 (2005)

101. Tariq, S M et al., The prevalence of and risk factors for atopy in early

childhood: A whole population birth cohort study, *J Allergy Clin Immunol*, vol 101, pp 587–593 (1998)

102. Tariq, S M *et al.* (1998)
103. Vally, H *et al.*, Alcoholic drinks: Important triggers for asthma, *J Allergy Clin Immunol*, vol 105, pp 462–7 (2000)
104. Butland, B K *et al.*, Diet, lung function, and lung function decline in a cohort of 2512 middle aged men, *Thorax*, vol 55, pp102–108 (2000)
105. Forastiere, F *et al.*, Consumption of fresh fruit rich in vitamin C and wheezing symptoms in children, *Thorax*, vol 55, pp 283–288 (2000)
106. Iack P *et al.*, *J Allergy Clin Immunol*, vol 103, pp 351–352 (1999)
107. Hodge, L *et al.*, Consumption of oily fish and childhood asthma, *Med J Aust*, vol 164, pp 137–140 (1996)
108. Kankaanpää, P *et al.*, Dietary fatty acids and allergy, *Ann Med*, vol 31, pp 282–287 (1999)
109. Soutar, A, Bronchial reactivity and dietary antioxidants,*Thorax*, vol 52, pp 166–170 (1997)
110. Mauskop, A *et al.*, Intravenous magnesium sulfate relieves migraine attacks in patents with low serum ionized magnesium levels: A pilot study, *Clin Sci*, vol 89, pp 633–636 (1995)
111. Trauninger, A *et al.*, Oral magnesium load test in patients with migraine, *Headache*, vol 42, pp 114–9 (2002)
112. Sprietsma, J E, Modern diets and diseases: NO-zinc balance. Under Th1, zinc and nitrogen monoxide (NO) collectively protect against viruses, AIDS, autoimmunity, diabetes, allergies, asthma, infectious diseases, atherosclerosis and cancer, *Med Hypotheses*, vol 53, pp 6–16 (1999)
113. Meloni, G *et al.*, Subclinical coeliac disease in school children from northern Sardinia, *The Lancet*, vol 353, p 37 (1999)
114. Mora, S *et al.*, Reversal of low bone density with a gluten-free diet in children and adolescents with celiac disease, *Am J Clin Nutr*, vol 67, pp 477–481 (1998)
115. Hoggan, R, Considering wheat, rye, and barley proteins as aids to carcinogens, *Med Hypotheses*, vol 49, pp 285–288 (1997)

Further Reading

Braly, J and Hoggan, R, *Dangerous Grains,* Penguin, 2003

Braly, J, *Food Allergy and Nutrition Revolution*, Keats, 1992

Holford, P, *Improve Your Digestion*, Piatkus, 1999

Holford, P, *New Optimum Nutrition Bible*, Piatkus, 2004

Holford, P, *Optimum Nutrition for the Mind*, Piatkus, 2003

Resources

■ Organisations and consultants

Allergy UK

Allergy UK is a charity supporting people with allergies or chemical sensitivity. Their website contains an abundance of information on allergies and products free of both food and non-food allergens. Visit www.allergyuk.org or call the Allergy Helpline +44 (0)1322 619864 or the Chemical Sensitivity Helpline +44 (0)1322 619898.

Brain Bio Centre

The Brain Bio Centre is an out-patient clinical treatment centre, specialising in the 'optimum nutrition' approach to mental health problems. The centre offers comprehensive assessment of biochemical imbalances such as food allergies that can contribute to mental health problems, and advice to correct these imbalances as a means to restore health. For more information visit www.brainbiocentre.com for a free downloadable information pack or call +44 (0)20 8871 9261.

British Society for Ecological Medicine

Formerly the British Society for Allergy, Environmental and Nutritional Medicine, this is the organisation for medical doctors working with allergies (including chemical sensitivities) and nutritional problems. Full members are all doctors; associate membership and other categories exist for related professions. The society holds regular meetings and publishes the *Journal of Nutritional and Environmental Medicine*. For further information (including a list of practitioners if needed) please write to PO Box 7, Knighton, Powys LD7 1WT, UK. Or call +44 (0)1547 550378, fax +44 (0)1547 550339, email info@bsaenm.org or call the information line +44 (0)906 3020010 (premium rates).

Institute for Optimum Nutrition (ION)

ION runs courses, including the Homestudy Course and the three-year Nutrition Therapy Foundation Degree Course (DipION/FdSc). It also has a directory of nutritional therapists throughout the UK. For details on courses, consultations and publications, contact ION at 13 Blades Court, Deodar Road, London SWI5 2NU. Or call +44 (0)20 8877 9993, fax +44 (0)20 8877 9980 or visit www.ion.ac.uk.

Nutrition consultations

For a personal referral by Patrick Holford to a nutritional therapist in your area, visit www.patrickholford.com and select 'consultations' for an immediate online referral. This service gives details on whom to see in the UK as well as internationally. If there is no one available nearby, you can always do an online assessment – see below.

Nutrition assessment online

You can have your own personal health and nutrition assessment online using the MyNutrition questionnaire. Visit www.patrick-holford.com and go to consultations.

Tests

In the UK

YORKTEST tests

YORKTEST's clinically proven foodSCAN range of food allergy tests using IgG ELISA testing could help you accurately identify your hidden food allergies from a list of 113 of the most common foods, and could bring relief from your symptoms. The test involves the collection of blood by a simple pin-prick, and laboratory analysis. For more information call 0800 074 6185 (a freephone number not available outside the UK), or visit www.yorktest.com. Also available are a classical IgE allergy test, and homocysteine test.

Intestinal permeability (leaky gut) test

This test is available from the following labs through qualified nutrition consultants and doctors:

- Biolab Medical Unit (doctor's referral only): call +44 (0)20 7636 5959

- Individual Well-being Diagnostic Laboratories: call +44 (0)20 8336 7750 or visit www.iwdl.net.

In Australia
ARL Pathology

Analytical Reference Laboratories (ARL) provides three IgG Food Sensitivity Tests. The most comprehensive of these, the IgG 93, tests for 93 different foods including wheat, dairy, eggs, soy and nuts. A blood sample is required and the test is suitable for all ages. For more information contact ARL free on 1300 55 44 80. You can email info@arlaus.com.au or visit www.arlaus.com for more details.

In South Africa
Molecular Diagnostic Services

Molecular Diagnostic Services offer IgG allergy testing for a wide range of foods, including a panel of 90 foods. They also have a self collection kit that enables you to take your own blood sample by a simple finger prick technique. For details telephone +27 31 267 1319, email mds@mdsafrica.net or visit www.mdsafrica.net.

Supplements and other products

Finding a supplement programme that's perfect for you can be confusing, but Patrick's website, www.patrickholford.com, offers useful guidance.

The backbone of a good supplement programme is:

- A high-strength multivitamin

- Additional vitamin C

- An all-round antioxidant complex

- An essential fat supplement containing omega-3 and omega-6 oils.

In this section we list some of our favourite herbal, food and nutritional supplements. The addresses of the companies whose products we've referred to are given at the end.

Useful herbal, food and nutritional supplements

Antioxidants

A good all-round antioxidant complex should provide vitamin A (beta-carotene and/or retinol), vitamins C and E, zinc, selenium, glutathione or cysteine, anthocyanidins of berry extracts, lipoic acid and co-enzyme Q10. Favourites are Higher Nature's AGE Antioxidant and Solgar's Advanced Antioxidant Nutrients. Complexes of bioflavonoids, often found together with vitamin C, are available from both companies. A good example is Solgar's Quercetin Complex which contains quercetin, bromelain and vitamin C. Higher Nature make an excellent range of MSM products, including creams and gels for topical use as well as MSM capsules, tablets and powders.

Digestive enzymes and support

Any decent digestive enzyme needs to contain enzymes to digest protein (protease), carbohydrate (amylase) and fat (lipase). Some also contain amyloglucosidase (also called glucoamylase), which digests glucosides founds in certain beans and vegetables noted for their flatulent effects. Our favourites are Solgar's Vegan Digestive Enzymes and Higher Nature's Supergest.

Some people have low levels of betaine hydrochloride (stomach acid). You can supplement this on its own and, if it helps digestion, then this may be your problem. Solgar's Digestive Aid supplement contains betaine HCL, plus other digestive enzymes. It is not vegetarian. Higher Nature do a 300mg supplement suitable for vegans.

Products for gut healing

Butyric acid and caprylic acid are triglycerides, or blood fats, that help to heal the gut wall, partly because the membranes of intestinal cells are largely made out of such fats. Biocare's Butyric Acid and Solgar's Caprylic Acid are both excellent. Higher Nature's Candiclear contains caprylic acid along with herbs that promote a healthy gut flora. Glutamine is an amino acid with gut-healing properties. Higher Nature make a very good glutamine powder in the most effective form.

Probiotics

Probiotics are supplements of beneficial bacteria, the two main strains being *Lactobacillus acidophilus* and *Bifidobacterium bifidus*. There are various types of strain within these two, some more important in children, others in adults. There is quite a lot of variability in amounts of bacteria (some labels say things like 'a billion viable organisms per capsule') and quality. We consider the following supplements to be high quality and well formulated: BioCare's Bifidoinfantis can be taken from birth to weaning; once weaned, babies and children can take BioCare's Banana or Strawberry Acidophilus powder, plain Bioacidophilus capsules or Solgar's ABCDophilus. Adults can try Higher Nature's Acidobifidus.

Essential fats and fish oil supplements

The most important omega-3 fats are DHA and EPA, the richest source being cod liver oil. The most important omega-6 fat is GLA, the richest source being borage or starflower oil. Try Higher Nature's Essential Omegas, which provides a highly concentrated mix of EPA, DHA and GLA. They also produce an Omega-3 Fish Oil supplement – good value, as is Seven Seas Extra High Strength Cod Liver Oil. Both these products have consistently proven the purest when tested for PCB residues, which are in almost all fish. Cod liver oil also contains vitamin A. Higher Nature's Starflower Oil and Solgar's One-A-Day GLA are good value if you only want omega-6 fats.

Get Up & Go!

This tasty breakfast shake that you can blend with milk, soya milk, rice milk or juice plus a banana or other fruit provides significant amounts of vitamins and minerals plus protein from a blend of rice, soya and quinoa, plus fibre from rice and oat bran, plus essential fatty acids from sesame, sunflower and pumpkin seeds. It has a delicious, totally natural flavour and contains no sucrose, additives, animal products, yeast, wheat or milk so it's a perfect breakfast if you're allergic to any of these. At less than 500 kcalories, this adds up to a substantial and sustaining healthy breakfast. Available from Higher Nature.

Multivitamin and mineral supplements

Supplementing the right multivitamin is the most important supplement decision you make. Most multivitamins are based on RDA levels of nutrients, which are not the same as optimum nutrition levels. The best multivitamin, based on optimum nutrition levels, is Higher Nature's Advanced Optimum

Nutrition Formula. The second best is Solgar's VM2000. Both of these recommend 2 tablets a day. Advanced Optimum Nutrition Formula has better mineral levels, especially for calcium and magnesium. Ideally, both should be taken with an extra 1g of vitamin C. Best of all is Higher Nature's Advanced Optimum Nutrition for Body and Mind Pack – a daily sachet of 2 multivitamins, 2 Immune Cs and 2 Essential Omegas.

Supplement suppliers

In the UK

The following companies produce good-quality supplements that are widely available in the UK.

BioCare Available in most health food shops. Call +44 (0)121 433 3727 or visit www.BioCare.co.uk.

Higher Nature Available in all good health food shops. Call +44 (0)845 3300012 for your nearest stockist, or visit www.highernature.co.uk.

Seven Seas Specialise in cod liver oil, rich in omega-3 fats. Available in health food shops and pharmacies. Visit www.sevenseas.ltd.uk.

Solgar Available in most health food shops. Call +44 (0)1442 890355 for your nearest supplier or visit www.solgar.co.uk.

Health Products for Life Offer a wide range of health products that we recommend, from supplements to air purifiers, by mail and online. But you can also order by calling +44 (0)20 8874 8038, or visit www.healthproductsforlife.com.

In other regions

South Africa Bioharmony produce a wide range of products in South Africa and other African countries. For details of your nearest supplier call 0860 888 339 or visit www.bioharmony. co.za.

Australia Solgar supplements are available in Australia. Call 1800 029 871 (freephone) for your nearest supplier or visit www. solgar.com.au. Another good brand available in Australia is Blackmores.

New Zealand Higher Nature products are available in New Zealand. Contact Aurora Natural Therapies, 445 Dillons Point Road, RD3, Blenheim, Marlborough, New Zealand, or visit www.Aurora.org.nz.

Singapore Higher Nature and Solgar products are available in Singapore. Please call Essential Living on 6276 1380 for your nearest supplier or visit www.essliv.com.

Skincare products

Environ products were developed by cosmetic surgeon Dr Des Fernandes to prevent skin cancer and address the damaging effects of the environment on our skin. Formulated with scientifically proven active ingredients including vitamin A and antioxidant vitamins C, E and beta-carotene, which are used in progressively higher concentrations, Environ helps to maintain a normal healthy skin, especially when there are signs of ageing, pigmentation, problem skin and scarring.

To purchase Environ products, call Health Products For Life on +44 (0)20 8874 8038, or go to www.healthproductsforlife. com. For international enquiries call +2721 683 1034, or go to environc@iafrica.com.

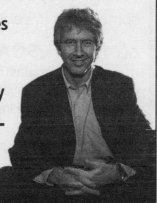

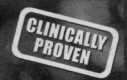
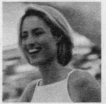

Index

(page numbers in italic type refer to illustrations)

THE HOLFORD LOW-GL DIET

Patrick Holford

Two simple rules
1. Eat no more than 40 GLs a day
2. Eat protein with carbohydrate

One simple diet
The Holford Low-GL Diet
At its heart, one controlling principle:
If you lose blood sugar control, you gain weight, and feel hungry and tired;
If you gain blood sugar control, you lose weight, feel happy and full of energy.

The bottom line
When you balance your blood sugar, you'll lose weight fast.

With *The Holford Low-GL Diet* you will beat your cravings! You'll enjoy delicious meals, choosing from a wide variety of energy-boosting foods and simple menu plans. The diet is safe and easy to follow, and includes a nutritional supplementation plan to increase your energy and decrease your appetite.

Tried and tested by the Institute for Optimum Nutrition, *The Holford Low-GL Diet* is based on the latest medical and nutritional research, made totally accessible. Discover how easy it is to reprogramme your body to burn your fat away.

£7.99
ISBN: 0 7499 2543 4

THE HOLFORD LOW-GL DIET COOKBOOK

Patrick Holford and Fiona McDonald Joyce

The Holford Low-GL Diet showed you how to lose fat fast, safely and permanently. It revealed how the key is to control the number of 'GLs' you consume each day. Based on the latest research, top nutritionist Patrick Holford explained that by eating no more than 40 GLs a day and eating protein with carbohydrate, you can lose weight quickly and permanently, control your blood sugar, improve your health and feel truly energised.

The Holford Low-GL Diet Cookbook is the perfect companion to *The Holford Low-GL Diet*. This attractively designed cookbook is packed with delicious tried-and-tested recipes which are both easy to follow and simple to prepare. The GLs of each recipe are clearly calculated for you, so it's easy to stick to your daily limit, especially with over 150 tempting recipes to choose from. With menu plans and recipes for both weight-loss and maintenance, *The Holford Low-GL Diet Cookbook* will enable you to beat cravings and lose weight permanently.

£12.99
ISBN: 0 7499 2642 2

PATRICK HOLFORD'S NEW OPTIMUM NUTRITION BIBLE

Patrick Holford

Completely revised and updated to include the latest cutting-edge research.

The bestselling *Optimum Nutrition Bible* has revolutionised health. It explains how, by giving yourself the best possible intake of nutrients, to allow your body to be as healthy as it possibly can. This revised and updated edition shows you:

- What a well balanced diet really means
- How to boost your immune system
- How to increase your energy and fitness levels
- How to prevent cancer and turn back the ageing clock
- How to avoid heart disease and lower your blood pressure without drugs
- Why the wrong fats can kill and the right fats can heal
- How to increase your IQ, memory and mental performance

Includes new charts and six new chapters, on Stimulants, Water, Eating right for your blood type, Detox, Homocysteine and Toxic Minerals.

£12.99
ISBN: 0 7499 2552 3

OPTIMUM NUTRITION FOR THE MIND

Patrick Holford

Optimum nutrition is a revolution in healthcare. Patrick Holford's first major book, *The Optimum Nutrition Bible*, dealt with the effect of good nutrition for the body. *Optimum Nutrition for the Mind* reveals what good nutrition can do for the mind. Some 80 per cent of us suffer from 'affluent malnutrition', and struggle to cope with the demands of 21st-century life. No wonder the World Health Organization has reported that mental health problems are fast becoming the world's number-one health issue.

This is the first definitive, readable and practical guide to solving mental health problems through nutrition. Read this book and find out how you can use optimum nutrition to:

- Increase your IQ and improve your concentration
- Boost your memory and sharpen your mind - whatever your age
- Improve your mood, banish mood swings and beat depression
- Conquer stress and anxiety and get a great night's sleep

And how optimum nutrition can:

- Reverse learning difficulties, dyslexia and hyperactivity
- Help children with Down's syndrome and autism
- Prevent and arrest dementia, Alzheimer's and Parkinson's disease
- Speed up recovery from schizophrenia

£12.99
ISBN: 0 7499 2398 9

THE ALZHEIMER'S PREVENTION PLAN

Patrick Holford with Shane Heaton and Deborah Colson

Alzheimer's disease and age-related memory loss are on the increase. The burden this places on sufferers, their families and health care systems is immense. In this reassuring and practical book, top nutritionist and mental health expert Patrick Holford argues that memory decline and Alzheimer's disease can be arrested and prevented and you *can* reduce your risks significantly if you take early action.

The Alzheimer's Prevention Plan is based on cutting-edge research into nutritional medicine from experts around the world. It contains a specially formulated Alzheimer's prevention diet and a ten-step plan to enhance your memory, which includes:

- A simple test to discover your risk – and reverse it in eight weeks
- Memory-boosting vitamins and minerals
- Essential fats that help your brain think faster
- Simple lifestyle changes and exercises to keep your mind young

£9.99
ISBN: 0 7499 2514 0

500 HEALTH AND NUTRITION QUESTIONS ANSWERED

Patrick Holford

In *500 Health and Nutrition Questions Answered* top nutritionist Patrick Holford answers a selection of the most important health questions he has been asked.

Armed with comprehensive knowledge of all things nutritional, he explains in simple, easy-to-follow terms the best way to deal with everything from common colds to unusual medical conditions, not forgetting those little complaints that you'd never take to your doctor. From how to prevent hangovers to nutritional tips for coping with skin conditions, depression, Alzheimer's, and Multiple Sclerosis, you'll find out what's good for you, what's not good for you – and why.

Includes sections on:

- Diet and nutrition, supplements and herbal remedies
- Diseases and common ailments
- Mental health
- Pregnancy, fertility and sex
- Energy and sleep, stress and fatigue
- Skin and hair
- Men's and women's health
- Weight loss
- And much more!

£8.99
ISBN: 0 7499 2493 4